Signals and Communication Technology

This series is devoted to fundamentals and applications of modern methods of signal processing and cutting-edge communication technologies. The main topics are information and signal theory, acoustical signal processing, image processing and multimedia systems, mobile and wireless communications, and computer and communication networks. Volumes in the series address researchers in academia and industrial R&D departments. The series is application-oriented. The level of presentation of each individual volume, however, depends on the subject and can range from practical to scientific.

Indexing: All books in "Signals and Communication Technology" are indexed by Scopus and zbMATH

For general information about this book series, comments or suggestions, please contact Mary James at mary.james@springer.com or Ramesh Nath Premnath at ramesh.premnath@springer.com.

Rohit Thanki • Sejal Shah

Artificial Intelligence for Early Detection and Diagnosis of Oral Cancer

Springer

Rohit Thanki
Senior IEEE Member
IEEE
Rajkot, Gujarat, India

Sejal Shah
Marwadi University
Rajkot, Gujarat, India

ISSN 1860-4862 ISSN 1860-4870 (electronic)
Signals and Communication Technology
ISBN 978-3-032-05055-7 ISBN 978-3-032-05056-4 (eBook)
https://doi.org/10.1007/978-3-032-05056-4

This Springer imprint is published by the registered company Springer Nature Switzerland AG
The registered company address is: Gewerbestrasse 11, 6330 Cham, Switzerland

Preface

Oral cancer remains a significant global health challenge, characterized by high morbidity and mortality rates, largely due to late-stage diagnoses. Despite advancements in medical science, the 5-year survival rate for oral cancer has seen only modest improvements over the past few decades, underscoring the urgent need for innovative approaches to early detection and diagnosis. It is within this critical context that the transformative potential of artificial intelligence (AI) emerges as a beacon of hope.

This book, *Artificial Intelligence for Early Detection and Diagnosis of Oral Cancer*, delves into the profound impact that AI technologies are having, and will continue to have, on revolutionizing the fight against this devastating disease. Traditionally, the diagnostic process for oral cancer has relied heavily on visual inspection and biopsy methods that, while foundational, can be subjective, time-consuming, and often detect the disease at advanced stages when treatment options are limited and prognoses are poorer.

Our aim in writing this book is to provide a comprehensive and insightful exploration of the current landscape and future directions of AI applications in oral cancer detection and diagnosis. We bring together diverse perspectives, from foundational AI concepts relevant to medical imaging to cutting-edge research in areas, such as convolutional neural networks for image analysis, natural language processing for clinical data interpretation, and predictive analytics for risk stratification. The chapters are meticulously crafted to offer both theoretical understanding and practical insights, making this work valuable for a broad audience.

This book is intended for clinicians, researchers, students, and technology developers who are interested in the intersection of AI and oral healthcare. Whether you are a dentist seeking to understand how AI can augment your diagnostic capabilities, a computer scientist looking to apply your expertise to real-world medical challenges, or a policymaker aiming to foster innovation in healthcare, we believe you will find this volume an indispensable resource.

It is our sincere hope that this book will not only inform and educate but also inspire further research and collaboration at the nexus of artificial intelligence and oral oncology. By harnessing the power of AI, we can collectively strive toward a future where oral cancer is detected earlier, treated more effectively, and its devastating impact on individuals and communities is significantly diminished. The journey ahead is promising, and we invite you to join us in exploring the transformative potential of AI in the early detection and diagnosis of oral cancer.

Overview of the Book

- **Chapter 1:** Discusses basic information about oral cancer, its prevalence, and the challenges in early detection.
- **Chapter 2:** Explores traditional diagnostic and treatment methods for oral cancer and their limitations.
- **Chapter 3:** Covers the foundational concepts of artificial intelligence, including various machine learning, deep learning, and computer vision algorithms, detailing their workings, advantages, and limitations in a healthcare context.
- **Chapter 4:**
  - Examines the role of AI and learning algorithms in healthcare, particularly in medical imaging for oral cancer.
  - Introduces and details specific deep learning models and their performance in the classification and analysis of oral lesions and images.
- **Chapter 5:**
  - Introduces a multimodal oral cancer assistant AI agent that utilizes both descriptive AI and generative AI for a comprehensive approach to oral cancer diagnosis and treatment.

Features of the Book

- Basic information about oral cancer and its diagnostic challenges.
- Detailed exploration of the transformative potential of AI in early detection and diagnosis of oral cancer.
- In-depth discussion of various AI learning algorithms, including machine learning, deep learning, and computer vision.
- Inclusion of specific AI models and techniques for analyzing medical images and clinical records related to oral cancer.

- Insights into the practical application of AI, including convolutional neural networks for image analysis, natural language processing for clinical data interpretation, and predictive analytics for risk stratification.
- Provide practical application of new AI approach based on descriptive AI and generative AI for oral cancer diagnosis and treatment.

Rajkot, India Rohit Thanki
Rajkot, India Sejal Shah

Competing Interests The authors have no competing interests to declare that are relevant to the content of this manuscript.

Acknowledgments

Our task has been made easier, and the final version of this book has been considerably improved, thanks to the support we have received. We extend our heartfelt thanks to the publishing team for their invaluable guidance and encouragement during the creation of this book. We also wish to thank our colleagues and peers for their insightful discussions and contributions that enriched the content.

Contents

List of Figures

List of Tables

Chapter 1
Introduction

1.1 Overview of Cancer

Cancer is a broad term for diseases characterized by uncontrolled cell growth with the potential to invade or spread to other parts of the body [1]. It has affected humans throughout recorded history. In fact, some of the earliest evidence of cancer comes from ancient Egypt: a papyrus dating to around 3000 BC describes cases of breast tumors treated by cauterization (burning), noting grimly that "there is no treatment" [2]. The word cancer itself originates from Hippocrates (460–370 BC), who used the term karkinos (Greek for crab) to describe tumors, likening the appearance of cut tumors with claw-like veins to a crab's shape [2]. For centuries, cancers were poorly understood and generally fatal. Progress in understanding cancer accelerated in the nineteenth century with the advent of modern pathology. Rudolf Virchow's work linking microscopic cellular abnormalities to disease laid the foundation for oncology as a scientific discipline. By the late nineteenth and early twentieth centuries, major treatment advances began to appear. The discovery of X-rays in 1895 by Wilhelm Roentgen led to the first uses of radiation therapy for cancer by the end of that decade [3]. Early chemotherapy drugs were introduced in the 1940s, for example, nitrogen mustard (derived from World War II chemical warfare research) was found to induce remission in lymphoma, marking the start of the chemotherapy era [4]. Over the twentieth century and into the twenty-first century, our knowledge of cancer biology expanded tremendously, leading to new treatment modalities and prevention strategies.

Cancer is usually multifactorial in origin, with both genetic and environmental contributors. Epidemiological research since the mid-twentieth century has identified many risk factors that increase the likelihood of developing cancer [5]. Most of these risk factors are related to lifestyle or environmental and are considered modifiable meaning that changes in behavior can reduce risk. Estimates by public health authorities suggest that between 30% and 50% of cancer deaths could be prevented

R. Thanki, S. Shah, *Artificial Intelligence for Early Detection and Diagnosis of Oral Cancer*, Signals and Communication Technology,
https://doi.org/10.1007/978-3-032-05056-4_1

by modifying or avoiding key risk factors [1]. Below are some of the major established risk factors for cancer:

- **Tobacco Use:** Tobacco smoking is the single largest risk factor in cancer worldwide. It is linked to cancers of the lung, oral cavity, larynx, esophagus, pancreas, bladder, and many others. Globally, tobacco exposure accounts for a substantial share of cancer cases and deaths in combination with alcohol. It was implicated in about 72% of head and neck cancer cases in one analysis [6].
- **Unhealthy and Obesity:** Dietary habits and nutritional status play an important role. Diets low in fruits and vegetables and high in processed or red meats have been to higher rates of cancers such as colorectal cancer [1]. Excess body weight and physical inactivity are also significant contributors to cancer including breast, colorectal, uterine, kidney, and among others [7].
- **Alcohol Consumption:** Heavy alcohol use is a major risk factor for certain cancers, particularly of the oral cavity, pharynx, larynx, esophagus, liver, and breast. While alcohol alone is carcinogenic, it synergizes strongly with tobacco, people who both smoke and drink have multiplicatively higher risks of cancers of the upper respiratory and digestive tracts [8].
- **Infectious Agents:** A significant percentage of cancers worldwide are caused by chronic infections. Oncogenic viruses are chief among these. For example, persistent infection with human papillomavirus (HPV) causes virtually all cervical cancers and a large fraction of oropharyngeal (throat) cancers, as well as anal and genital cancers.
- **Radiation Exposure:** Exposure to ionizing radiation can induce DNA mutations that lead to cancer. Survivors of atomic bombs and nuclear accidents have higher rates of leukemia, thyroid cancer, and others. Medical use of radiation is kept as low as reasonably possible to balance diagnostic/treatment benefits against cancer risk.
- **Environmental and Occupational Carcinogens:** Various chemicals and pollutants can cause cancer with chronic exposure. Examples include asbestos (mesothelioma and lung cancer), benzene (leukemia), arsenic (skin, lung, and bladder cancer), certain dyes and industrial chemicals, and air pollution. Notably, ambient air pollution has been identified as one of the top five contributors to global cancer burden [7].
- **Age and Genetic Factors:** Simply getting order is a risk factor for cancer, as mutations accumulate over time. Most cancers occur in people over 50. Family history and genetics also play a role, and small percentages of cancers are highly influenced by inherited gene mutations. Individuals with strong family histories may benefit from genetic counseling and earlier screening.

Cancers are classified based on their primary site (initial location) and histological type (tissue of origin). The first method is categorizing cancer by histological type. The International Classification of Diseases for Oncology, Third Edition (ICD-O-3), is the global standard for this classification. There are hundreds of histologically distinct cancers, grouped into six main categories [9].

- **Carcinoma:** Carcinomas are cancers starting in epithelial tissue, making up 80–90% of cases. They include squamous cell carcinomas from squamous epithelium and adenocarcinomas from glandular tissues, often affecting organs like the breast, colon, and lungs.
- **Sarcoma:** A cancer originating in connective tissues such as muscle, fat, cartilage, and tendons. Common types include osteosarcoma (bones), chondrosarcoma (cartilage), leiomyosarcoma (smooth muscle), and rhabdomyosarcoma (skeletal muscle).
- **Myeloma:** Myeloma is a kind of cancer that starts in the plasma cells of the bone marrow. Plasma cells produce a fraction of the proteins found in the blood.
- **Leukemia:** Leukemia is a blood cancer affecting bone marrow, resulting in abnormal production of immature white blood cells, causing infection risks, anemia, and fatigue. It includes myelogenous and lymphocytic types, with polycythemia vera affecting red blood cells.
- **Lymphoma:** Lymphomas arise in the lymphatic system, which includes the tonsils, thymus, and spleen. They are categorized as Hodgkin or non-Hodgkin lymphoma based on the presence of Reed–Sternberg cells.
- **Mixed Types:** The type components may be within one category or from different categories. Some examples are adenosquamous carcinoma, mixed mesodermal tumor, carcinosarcoma, etc.

Diagnosing cancer is a multifaceted process that requires a thorough medical history, physical examinations, and specialized diagnostic tests. Numerous tests are often necessary to distinguish cancer symptoms from those of other illnesses. Effective diagnostic procedures help confirm the presence or absence of the disease, monitor its progression, and evaluate the effectiveness of treatments. Occasionally, repeated testing may be needed due to changes in the condition, inadequate sample quality, or unusual test results. Common diagnostic methods include imaging, laboratory tests, tumor biopsies, endoscopic examinations, surgical procedures, and genetic testing. These approaches collectively aid in pinpointing the nature of cancer and tailoring the treatment strategy. The diagnostic methods used for cancer are as follows: laboratory tests, diagnostic imaging, endoscopic examinations, genetic testing, and tumor biopsies.

With the introduction of new tools and methods that can both help patients avoid surgery and more accurately diagnosed cancer, diagnostic radiography has evolved significantly in recent years. The doctors and diagnostic radiology personnel at Stanford Cancer Center are among the leading professionals in their industry, and they have access to advanced cancer imaging technologies available on the market. Due to the high regard for our doctors' expertise, we function as a reference center for other physicians, who may submit complex or borderline images to be expertly interpreted for their patients. The Cancer Center was built with state-of-the-art equipment and skilled personnel to enhance the quality of diagnostic radiological services [10].

Imaging is a crucial process for detecting tumors, determining disease extent, and evaluating treatment effectiveness. Emission, transmission, and reflection imaging are the three imaging modalities used in the diagnosis of cancer. By generating high-energy photons, transmission imaging creates a darker region on the X-ray film that passes through the body structure being inspected [11, 12]. High-frequency sounds are applied to the body part or organ under study during reflection imaging, and they bounce off different tissues and structures at different rates. A computer then analyzes these sound waves to create a graphic representation of the body component or structure. An additional imaging method for the diagnosis of cancer is ultrasound. When microscopic nuclear particles or magnetic energy are picked up by a scanner and processed by a computer, it creates a picture of the organ or body part under investigation. This process is known as emission imaging. Emission of radioactive particles from nuclear substances injected into the body expressly for the purpose of inspection is used in nuclear medicine. A device that generates a high magnetic field and utilizes radio waves to cause cells to produce their own radio frequencies is called a magnetic resonance imaging (MRI) machine [12, 13]. Cystoscopy, colonoscopy, esophagogastroduodenoscopy, endoscopic retrograde cholangiopancreatography (ERCP), and sigmoidoscopy are among the endoscopic exams used to identify malignancy. Understanding these concepts is crucial when considering cancer susceptibility gene testing since genetic testing for mutations in genes that promote cancer susceptibility is a complex process [14, 15]. Tumor biopsies are procedures carried out to take tissue or cells out of the body for microscopic inspection. Endoscopic, bone marrow, incisional or excisional, punch, shave, fine needle aspiration, and skin biopsies are examples of common forms.

Cancer is a global health issue causing one in six deaths. Traditional treatments include surgery, chemotherapy, and radiotherapy. Recent advancements involve radionics, chemo dynamic treatment, sonodynamic therapy, targeted therapy, ablation therapy, nanoparticles, natural antioxidants, and ferroptosis-based therapy. Modern oncology aims to develop effective and safe cancer nanomedicines. Nanoparticles offer new opportunities for diagnosis and treatment, while stem cell therapy shows promise for tissue regeneration and repair. Targeted therapies aim to stop cancer cell growth and spread with minimal damage to healthy cells. Ablation therapy offers a less invasive method to destroy tumors. Natural antioxidants combat free radicals.

Conventional cancer treatments like surgery, radiotherapy, and chemotherapy have limitations such as damaging healthy cells, drug resistance, and side effects. Despite these challenges, recognized therapeutic modalities and medications exist. Tumor pathology and abnormal blood vessel features decrease conventional treatment effectiveness. Surgery aims to remove as much cancer as possible. Chemotherapy uses drugs to kill cancer cells. Radiation therapy employs high-energy beams to target cancer cells. Bone marrow transplants increase chemotherapy doses. Immunotherapy boosts the body's defenses against cancer by helping the immune system recognize and fight it. Hormone therapy targets cancers fueled by body hormones, such as breast and prostate cancer. Targeted drug therapy focuses on specific cancer flaws. Radiofrequency ablation uses electrical energy to heat and kill cancer cells. Clinical trials explore new cancer treatments.

Targeted medicine enhances the distribution of chemotherapeutic drugs around treated tissues. Gene therapy introduces foreign genes into benign tumors. Stem cells contribute to immune cell generation, medication targeting, regenerative medicine, and therapeutic carriers. Thermal ablation and magnetic hyperthermia present alternatives to growth surgery. Radionics and pathomics techniques manage large datasets from cancer patients to improve prognosis and outcomes.

1.2 Oral Anatomy

To understand oral cancer, it is essential to be familiar with the basic anatomy of the oral cavity. The oral cavity (mouth) encompasses the structures at the beginning of the digestive tract and is delineated by several boundaries. It is bounded anteriorly by the lips, laterally by the cheeks, superiorly by the hard palate (the bony front part of the roof of the mouth), inferiorly by the floor of the mouth (under the tongue), and posteriorly it transitions into the oropharynx (the throat area behind the mouth) at a region roughly defined by the back of the tongue and the soft palate [16]. The bony foundations of the oral cavity are the maxilla (upper jaw) and mandible (lower jaw), which house the teeth. Key structures within the oral cavity include the following [16] (as shown in Fig. 1.1):

- The lips (external muscular folds that guard the mouth opening).
- The gingivae or gums (the soft tissue covering the jaw bones around the teeth).
- The teeth (embedded in the sockets of the maxilla and mandible, involved in biting and chewing).

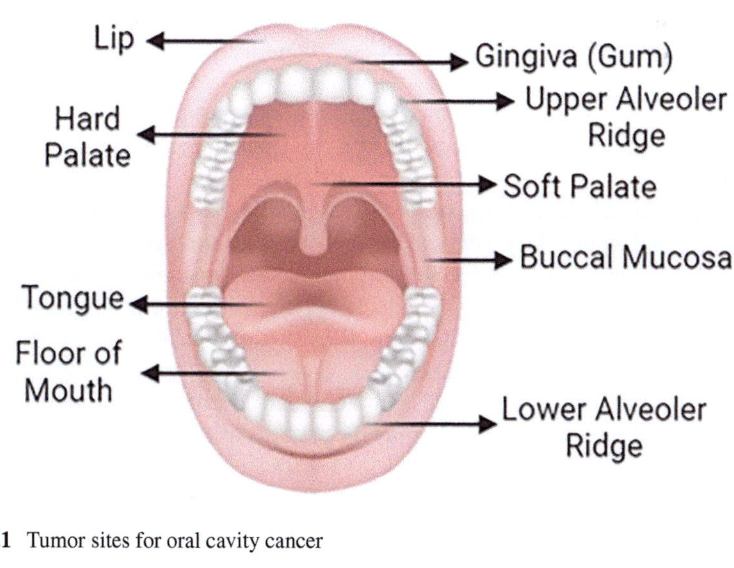

Fig. 1.1 Tumor sites for oral cavity cancer

- The tongue: specifically the front two-thirds of the tongue, which lies in the mouth (often called the oral tongue or mobile tongue). The tongue's back one-third (base of tongue) belongs to the oropharynx, not the oral cavity.
- The floor of the mouth: the region underneath the tongue, a common site for oral cancers.
- The buccal mucosa (the inner lining of the cheeks and inner aspect of the lips).
- The hard palate: the front part of the roof of the mouth, which is bony. (The soft palate is the rear part of the roof of the mouth and is considered part of the oropharynx.)
- The retromolar trigone: a small area of mucosa behind the last molar teeth on each side, bridging between the lower jaw and the throat.
- The oral vestibule: the space between the cheeks/lips and the teeth, which is technically part of the oral cavity (it's the area where you place your toothbrush or where chewing tobacco might sit in the cheek).

Just beyond the oral cavity, the oropharynx includes the soft palate, the tonsils, the base of tongue, and the back wall of the throat. These distinctions are important because cancers in the oral cavity versus the oropharynx have somewhat different risk factors and clinical behaviors (for example, HPV-related cancers often arise in the oropharynx, not the oral cavity proper).

Additionally, the mouth contains many minor salivary glands scattered beneath the mucosal lining (for instance, in the lips and palate). The major salivary glands the parotid, submandibular, and sublingual glands are located adjacent to the oral cavity and secrete saliva into it, but by anatomical definition, those glands themselves are considered separate from the oral cavity structures. Still, they are in proximity, and cancers of the salivary glands are another category of head and neck cancers (distinct from oral cavity cancer).

A rich network of blood vessels and nerves supplies the oral cavity. For example, the external carotid artery via the lingual and facial branches provides blood supply, and sensation is provided by branches of the trigeminal nerve (cranial nerve V) for most of the mucosa, while taste in the tongue involves the facial nerve (VII) for the anterior tongue. Muscles such as the tongue muscles and floor of mouth muscles (mylohyoid, etc.) form the functional anatomy enabling speech, chewing, and swallowing.

The lymphatic drainage of the oral cavity primarily flows to the submental, submandibular, and upper deep cervical lymph nodes in the neck. This is relevant because oral cancers can spread to those lymph nodes. In summary, the oral cavity contains numerous structures any of which can be a site of origin for oral cancer. Understanding these anatomical sites (lips, tongue, gums, palate, etc.) helps in identifying where an oral cancer is located and determining appropriate treatment (since, for instance, a cancer on the tongue may be managed differently than one on the hard palate). The anatomy also underpins the patterns of spread of oral cancer, both locally and to lymph nodes.

1.3 What Is Oral Cancer?

After cardiovascular diseases, cancer is the second leading cause of death worldwide [17]. One definition of cancer is a pathological state in which a collection of abnormal cells proliferates unchecked, disregarding the normal rules guiding cell division. Signals control the course of normally functioning cells when get disturbed; hence, cancer cells become independent and proliferate out of control. If permitted to spread, this proliferation might be lethal. Approximately, 90% of cancer-related deaths are caused by tumor metastases [18]. Urbanization, industrialization, changes in lifestyle (smoking, bad diet, lack of physical activity, and reproductive changes), population growth, genetics, and aging have all contributed to the global epidemiological shift of cancer [19]. Unfortunately, attempts to reduce incidence and mortality rates from cancer are not meeting their full potential, particularly in low-income countries [20]. The "cancer divide," which has worse results and a large burden among socioeconomically disadvantaged people, has drawn attention from the international health community, which has concentrated on global oncology. However, there is hope that cancer survival rates will rise dramatically because of recent developments in personalized medicine and cutting-edge therapeutic approaches like immunotherapy [21].

Oral cancer is the blazing dilemma globally. Oral cancer is the subset of HNSCC (head and neck squamous cell carcinoma) comprising almost all head and neck cancer categories. There are two types of oral cancers such as oral squamous cell carcinoma (OSCC) and oral basal cell carcinoma. OSCC accounts for approximately 90% of the oral cancers [22]. Different subsites of oral cavity cancers include buccal mucosa, palatal region, upper and lower gum, alveolar ridge, retromolar trigone, oropharynx (the middle portion of the esophagus connects to the oral cavity), floor of mouth, and lip mucosa [23] (as shown in Fig. 1.1).

Tumor progression starts from the regional to cervical lymph node in case of oral cancer. The cancer or tumor classification is inclined by the size of the tumor, site of the lymph node covered, and invasion sites of the tumor for cancer staging [24]. Oral squamous cell carcinoma (OSCC) is the most frequent form of oral cancer, accounting for nearly 90% of reported oral malignancies [25]. The spread of OSCC to the regional lymph nodes is the most important factor in determining the prognosis and treatment. Therefore, early diagnosis and prompt treatment are essential for successful outcomes. Early diagnosis is usually achieved through physical examination and imaging tests. Treatment options include surgery, radiation, and chemotherapy. Early diagnosis of OSCC significantly improves the chances of successful treatment and can greatly enhance the patient's quality of life. Detecting cancer at an initial stage often means less invasive treatment options and a higher likelihood of complete remission. Moreover, early intervention can prevent cancer from spreading to other areas, reducing the risk of complications and improving overall survival rates. Therefore, regular check-ups and early detection are essential for successful treatment of OSCC.

1.4 Incidence, Prevalence, and Mortality of Oral Cancer

Several cancer registries around the world provide statistics on cancer. A cancer registry data enlightens us on the prevalence of cancer, etiology research, early diagnosis as well as the accomplishment of various cancer-control initiatives. The two well-established online cancer databases are Global Cancer Observatory (GLOBOCAN) and Global Burden of Disease (GBD) offered by the International Agency for Research on Cancer (IARC) and the Institute for Health Metrics and Evaluation (IHME), respectively [26]. According to recent estimates, oral cancer is the 16th most prevalent cancer out of 36 cancers in the world which accounts for annual incidence of 389,765 (2% of all sites) cases and a mortality rate of 188, 438 (1.8% all sites) in 2022 [27] (as shown in Fig. 1.2).

According to the World Health Organization (WHO) [1], incidence refers to the occurrence rate of new cases in a specific population over a given period. The estimated age-standardized incidence rate (ASR) (W) of oral and lip cancer for both sexes is 4.0 per 100,000 people among all malignancies worldwide (as shown in

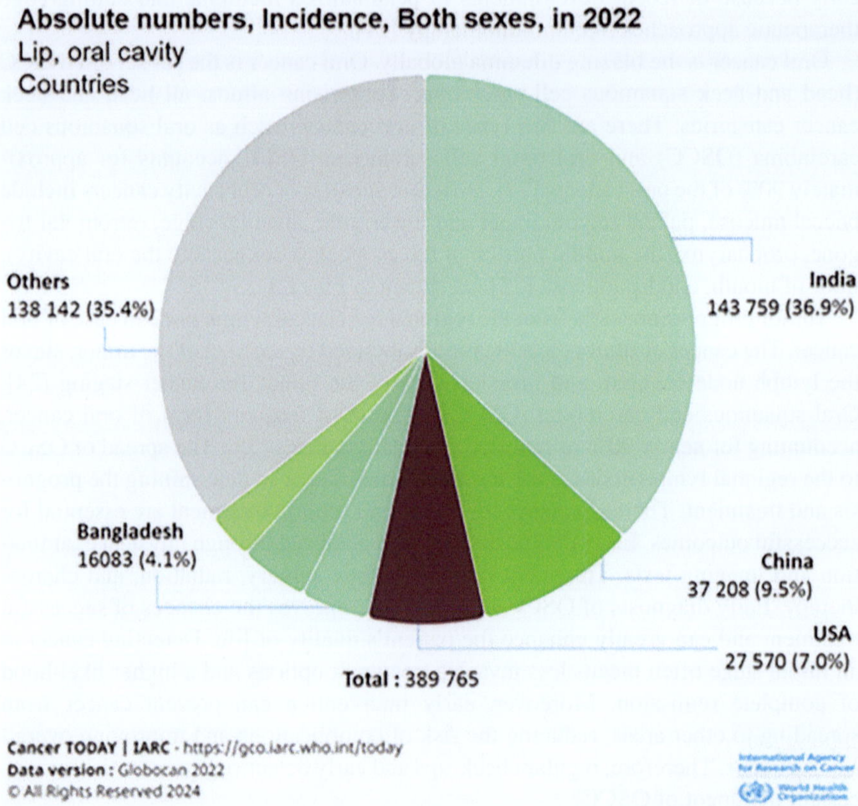

Fig. 1.2 Estimated number of new cases of oral cancer in the world (GLOBOCAN 2022, [28])

Fig. 1.3). The mortality rate is the frequency of oral cancer deaths among a specified population during a predetermined time, as defined by the WHO. In addition to a high incidence rate, a high death rate (5.6 per 100,000 ASR) was also reported in the Indian population compared to the global average (1.9 per 100,000 ASR) (as shown in Fig. 1.4).

India bears a significant portion of the global oral cancer burden [30]. According to the National Cancer Registry Program (NCRP) report (NCRP 2020), lip and oral

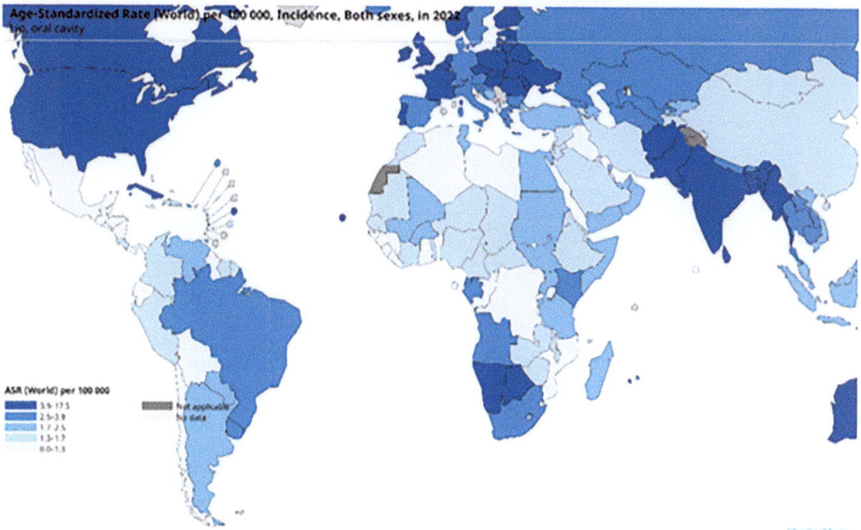

Fig. 1.3 The global incidence of oral cancer (GLOBOCAN 2022, [28])

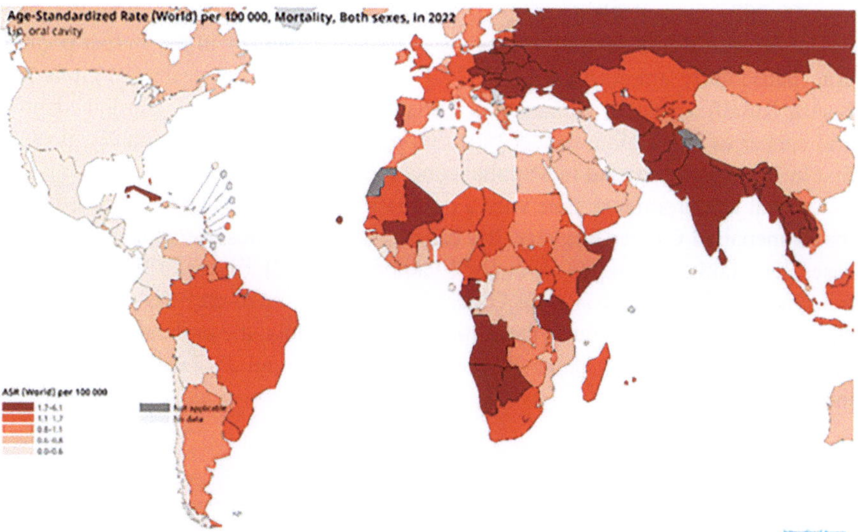

Fig. 1.4 The global mortality rate of oral cancer (GLOBOCAN 2022, [28])

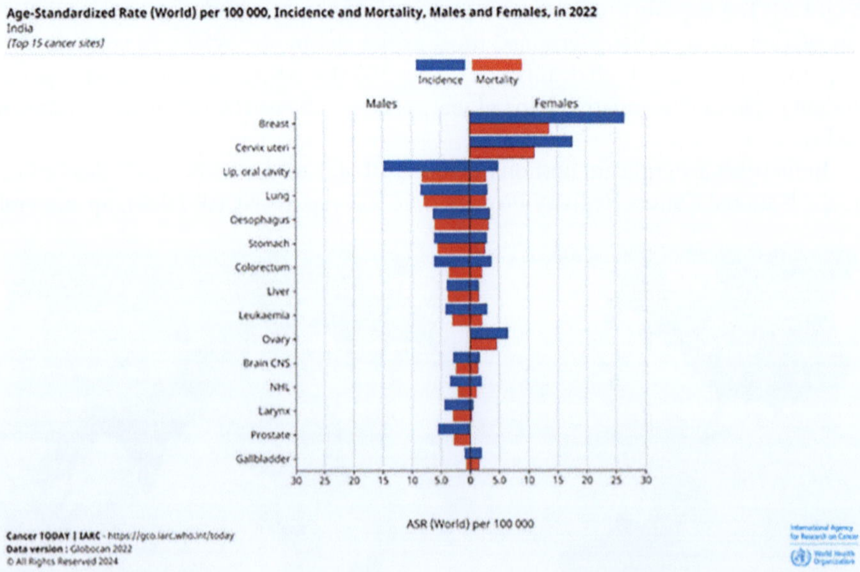

Fig. 1.5 Estimated ASR (W) of incidence and mortality rate of oral cancer in Indian male and female population [28]

cancer rank as the most prevalent cancer among Indian men, with an incidence and mortality age-standardized rate (ASR (W)) of 14.7 and 8.2 per 100,000, respectively. Comparatively, this cancer type ranks 16th globally among all cancers. For Indian women, oral cancer is the fourth most common type, following breast, cervical, and ovarian cancers, with an incidence and mortality ASR (W) of 5.0 and 2.9 per 100,000, respectively (as shown in Fig. 1.5). These statistics show that oral cancer incidence and mortality rates are significantly higher in the Indian population, particularly among men [31, 32]. Cancer registries in western regions like Barshi Rural/Expanded, Ahmedabad Urban, Nagpur, Pune, and Wardha identify oral cancer as the leading cancer type among male patients. Additionally, it ranks first in Bhopal and second in Mumbai cancer registries.

Gujarat is a prominent state with a population exceeding 6 crores. According to the Ahmedabad Cancer Registry, the cancer incidence rates are approximately 98 cases per 1 lakh men and 78 cases per 1 lakh women [32]. Figures 1.6 and 1.7 illustrate the top five cancer sites in Gujarati men and women and the percentage of cancers linked to tobacco use, respectively [33]. Notably, the oral cancer incidence rate in the Ahmedabad Cancer Registry stands at around 28.7 cases per 100,000 individuals [29].

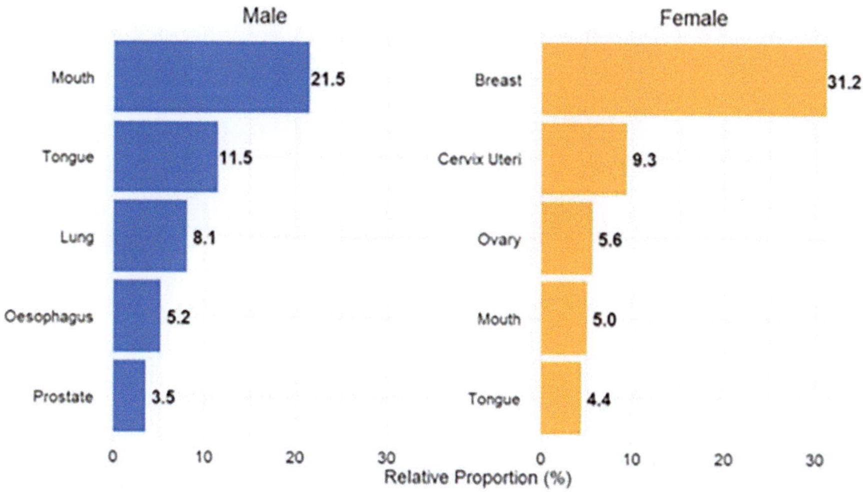

Fig. 1.6 Leading anatomical sites of cancer in Gujarati population [32]

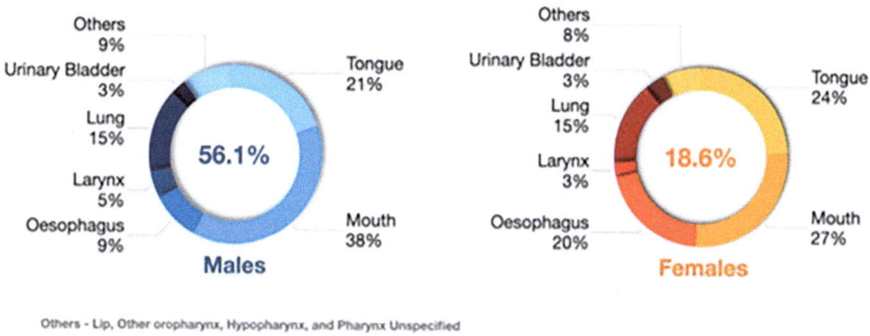

Fig. 1.7 Proportion (%) of cancer sites associated with the use of tobacco [32]

1.5 Risk Factors for Oral Cancer

Oral cancer diagnoses are climbing to new heights every single day. According to the International Agency for Research on Cancer (IARC, Cancer Tomorrow), the number of oral cancer patients in India is projected to reach approximately 209,169 (a 53% increase) by the year 2040. Consequently, there is a pressing need to narrow down the management of patients with oral cancer. The primary causes of OSCC are tobacco chewing, snuffing, smoking bidis, gutkha, betel nuts, alcohol intake, and human papillomavirus (HPV) infection (as shown Fig. 1.8) [34, 35].

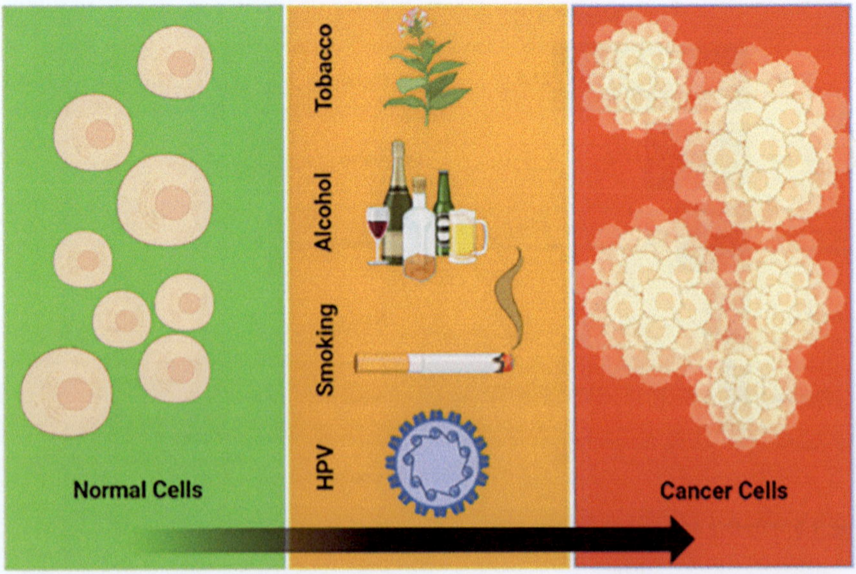

Fig. 1.8 Major risk factors developing oral cancer (exposure to carcinogenic agents such as cigarettes, alcohol, smoking, and human papillomavirus can transform normal cells into cancerous cells)

1.5.1 Tobacco Smoking and Chewing

It is well documented that tobacco smoking and chewing are significant risk factors for the development of oral cancer. The primary methods of tobacco consumption include chewing tobacco products, smoking, and inhalation. Tobacco is derived from the plants Nicotiana tabacum and Nicotiana rustica. These plants contain the volatile alkaloid nicotine in their leaves, which binds to central nervous system receptors and elevates dopamine levels, resulting in addiction [36]. Tobacco contains over 5000 chemicals or compounds that are toxic and carcinogenic [37]. Numerous carcinogenic chemical compounds, including N′-nitrosonornicotine (NNN), N-nitrosamines (TSNA), and polycyclic aromatic hydrocarbon (PAH), have been identified in smokeless tobacco products [38]. The use of smokeless tobacco (SLT) in forms such as betel quid (pan) and betel quid substitutes (pan masala, gutkha, mawa), oral snuff (Masheri, Gul, Gudhaku), and chewing tobacco (Khaini, Zarda, Kimam) can increase the risk of oral squamous cell carcinoma (OSCC) by 2 to 15 times [39].

In addition to oral cancer, tobacco smoking is linked to lung, larynx, esophageal, and other types of cancer. Common ways to smoke tobacco include cigarettes, cigars, pipes, and traditional Middle Eastern bidis. Hookahs and chillums, clay pipes used to keep burning tobacco, are popular in India and some other Asian countries [40]. Compared to cigarettes, the unprocessed tobacco used in bidis has been shown to increase the risk of cancer [41].

In the Asia and Pacific region, betel quid chewing is a common practice, with approximately 10% of the global population regularly engaging in this activity [42]. The Indian market is inundated with low-quality products containing betel nut, tobacco, and various spice items. These commodities are rich in Reactive Oxygen Species (ROS), catechu polyphenols, and slaked lime content. Depending on ROS production levels, oxidative stress, and ROS formation may trigger cell growth, senescence, or even apoptosis. Prolonged exposure to these mutagens can result in oral mucosal ulcers and eventually cancer [43].

Smokeless tobacco products account for more than 50% of Oral Squamous Cell Carcinoma (OSCC) diagnoses in India [44]. Previous studies have documented that chewing tobacco can lead to OSCC development by activating the nuclear factor-kB (NF-κB) and signal transducer and activator of transcription 3 (STAT-3) pathways [45, 46]. To combat the rising popularity of tobacco products, the government has mandated the inclusion of pictorial and textual health warning labels (HWL) on cigarette and gutkha packages [47, 48].

1.5.2 Alcohol

The consumption of alcoholic beverages is a significant contributor to the global prevalence of oral squamous cell carcinoma (OSCC) [49]. In conjunction with other carcinogens, alcohol may have an additive effect in the development of cancers of the oral cavity, larynx, and esophagus. Research indicates that alcohol may facilitate the uptake of carcinogens by oral mucosal cells, potentially leading to cancer [50]. Studies have shown that individuals who consume more than 170 grams of whisky daily have a tenfold increased risk of developing ovarian cancer compared to light drinkers [51].

In addition to known carcinogens such as N-nitroso compounds, acetaldehyde, the primary metabolite of alcohol, is produced from ethanol by the enzyme alcohol dehydrogenase (ADH). Acetaldehyde was classified as a carcinogen by the International Agency for Research on Cancer (IARC) in 1999, and in 2009, it was further classified as a Group 1 carcinogen for humans [52]. Acetaldehyde damages DNA and inhibits its replication and repair by blocking 6-methylguanine-DNA methyltransferase, an enzyme essential for repairing DNA errors caused by alkylating agents. This process also triggers sister chromatid exchanges and targeted gene alterations [53].

However, current evidence does not suggest that pure ethanol alone is a carcinogen for the onset of oral cancer. It is widely recognized that the combination of alcohol and tobacco has a synergistic effect that significantly increases the risk of cancer.

1.5.3 *Human Papillomavirus (HPV)*

Many oncogenic viruses significantly contribute to human malignancies. The double-stranded DNA virus HPV is most frequently linked with oropharyngeal cancer (OC) [54]. HPV is a potential risk factor for head and neck squamous cell carcinoma (HNSCC), especially from the oropharynx [55], primarily transmitted through oral sexual activity [56]. HPV-16 is found in 90–95% of HPV-positive HNSCC cases, followed by HPV-18, HPV-31, HPV-33, HPV-35, and HPV-39. The HPV genome encodes E6 and E7 proteins, which attach to tumor suppressor genes P53 and Rb, disrupting their roles in the cell cycle, replication, repair, and apoptosis pathways [57]. The prevalence of HPV in Asian OSCC is higher compared to other regions [58].

1.6 Prevention Against Oral Cancer

Most oral cancers are linked to modifiable habits, making prevention feasible and crucial. It is largely preventable as the main risk factors are known and can be reduced or eliminated [59]. Effective prevention includes public health measures, individual lifestyle changes, and medical interventions to detect and treat precancerous conditions. Key strategies for preventing oral cancer are:

- **Tobacco Cessation and Avoidance:** Quitting tobacco use is essential to prevent oral cancer. This includes stopping cigarette smoking and avoiding smokeless tobacco. Public health policies like tobacco taxes, warning labels, advertising bans, and smoke-free laws, along with cessation support (counseling, nicotine replacement therapy, medications) can significantly reduce smoking rates. In high-risk areas, it's crucial to address betel quid chewing through education and support to quit. Former users see a decline in oral cancer risk within years of quitting, though it may not match that of non-users. Avoiding second-hand smoke is also important as it can increase oral and throat cancer risks in non-smokers.
- **Limiting Alcohol Consumption:** Moderation of alcohol intake, or abstaining altogether, is important for oral cancer prevention. For those who drink, it is advised to stay within the recommended limits (e.g., no more than one drink per day for women or two for men, according to many health guidelines). Public health initiatives to reduce alcohol abuse, such as excise taxes, drinking-and-driving enforcement, and treatment programs for alcohol dependence, can benefit communities with prevalent heavy drinking. Combining alcohol reduction with tobacco cessation provides the greatest risk reduction. Individuals who both smoke and drink should be informed that quitting both is crucial, as stopping only one still leaves significant risk due to the synergistic effect.
- **Protective Diet and Nutrition:** A diet rich in fruits, vegetables, and whole food provides antioxidants and micronutrients that protect oral tissues. To increase

fresh produce intake, focus on especially leafy greens and foods high in vitamins A, C, and E. Avoid diets high in salted or preserved foods. Nutritional supplements and education can reduce cancer risk in malnourished populations. Clinical trials on antioxidant vitamins for oral precancer prevention show mixed results, but a balanced diet supports overall health and lowers cancer risk. Staying hydrated and maintaining good general health also support mucosal integrity.

- **Oral Hygiene and Dental Care:** Good oral hygiene and regular dental check-ups help prevent or detect oral cancer early. Chronic, flossing, and addressing chronic dental issues like sharp tooth edges and ill-fitting dentures can reduce cancer risk. Dentists can screen for oral cancer during routine visits. Public awareness encourages seeing a dentist if mouth ulcers or patches persist for over 2 weeks. Early treatment of precancerous lesions can prevent invasive cancer.
- **HPV Vaccination:** While HPV is not a major cause of oral cavity cancer, it is linked to many oropharyngeal cancers. Vaccinating adolescents (both girls and boys) can reduce HPV infections that lead to cervical and other cancers. Widespread HPV vaccination may decrease HPV-associated head and neck cancers over time [8]. Although its direct impact on oral cavity cancer is unclear, HPV vaccination is recommended as a general cancer preventive measure. It is safe and effective, ideally given before sexual activity begins. Countries with HPV vaccination programs have seen declines in cervical and some oropharyngeal cancers, indicating a positive trend for the future.
- **UV Protection for Lips:** To prevent lip cancer, especially for outdoor workers, use SPF lip balms, wear broad-brimmed hats, and avoid peak UV exposure. This is like skin cancer prevention. Those with fair skin or a history of lip damage should be extra cautious.
- **Avoidance of Other Carcinogens:** Reducing exposure to environmental or workplace carcinogens is crucial. Workplace safety for handling chemicals like asbestos or heavy metals lowers cancer risks, including oral cancers. Overall, a healthy environment with clean air and water aids in cancer prevention.
- **Awareness and Early Detection (Secondary Prevention):** Despite primary prevention, some will develop precancerous changes or early cancers. Educating the public and healthcare providers about early signs of oral cancer is crucial. Key symptoms include a non-healing mouth sore, cheek lump, white or red patches on gums or tongue, difficulty swallowing or moving the jaw, unexplained mouth bleeding or numbness, and persistent ear pain. Immediate evaluation is necessary if these occur.
- Regular dental exams often function as oral cancer screenings, allowing dentists to detect suspicious lesions and refer patients for biopsies. Some countries have implemented population screening in high-risk groups, such as mobile clinics in India targeting tobacco chewers. Targeted screening of high-risk individuals (e.g., long-term smokers and drinkers) improves early detection rates. A randomized trial in India showed that visual oral exams by health workers led to earlier cancer detection and reduced mortality in high-risk populations.
- Routine population-wide screening isn't cost-effective for oral cancer, but opportunistic screening during dental or medical visits is highly encouraged. Early

detection serves as secondary prevention because treating precancers or early cancers can prevent lethal advanced cancers.

- **Treatment of Precancerous Lesions:** Identifying precancerous lesions (such as leukoplakia, erythroplakia, or submucous fibrosis) calls for preventive management. This may involve surgical removal, laser ablation, or close monitoring with risk habit advice. Some disorders have high transformation rates (e.g., erythroplakia often shows high-grade dysplasia), so removing them or using adjunctive therapies like retinoids can prevent carcinoma [59]. Regular follow-ups are necessary for patients with such lesions.

Public health efforts to prevent oral cancer focus on education and awareness. These include anti-tobacco and anti-alcohol campaigns, school programs warning against betel nut chewing, and training primary healthcare workers for oral exams. Community outreach is vital, especially in rural areas or among lower socioeconomic groups at higher risk.

In summary, preventing oral cancer involves addressing its root causes (tobacco, alcohol, betel, etc.) and promoting early detection. The World Health Organization notes that comprehensive tobacco control alone could drastically reduce not only oral cancer but also many other cancers [1]. Likewise, ensuring that people have access to dental care and encouraging healthy lifestyles contributes to lowering oral cancer incidence. Despite these efforts, one challenge is that the incidence of oral cancer has not declined as much in some regions, partly due to entrenched cultural habits like betel chewing and the lag in behavior change. Therefore, continued and culturally appropriate prevention strategies are needed. With concerted efforts, oral cancer can be significantly curtailed, improving public health outcomes and reducing the burden of this often-devastating disease [59].

References

1. *Cancer*. Retrieved April 2025, from https://www.who.int/health-topics/cancer#tab=tab_1
2. *Understanding what cancer is: Ancient times to present*. Retrieved April 2025, from https://www.cancer.org/cancer/understanding-cancer/history-of-cancer/what-is-cancer.html#:~:text=Some%20of%20the%20earliest%20evidence,neck%20has%20been%20found%2C%20too
3. *History of cancer treatments: Radiation therapy*. Retrieved April 2025, from https://www.cancer.org/cancer/understanding-cancer/history-of-cancer/cancer-treatment-radiation.html#:~:text=In%201896%20a%20German%20physics,used%20in%20to%20treat%20cancer
4. *History of cancer treatments: Chemotheraphy*. Retrieved April 2025, from https://www.cancer.org/cancer/understanding-cancer/history-of-cancer/cancer-treatment-chemo.html#:~:text=During%20World%20War%20II%2C%20naval,cells%20by%20damaging%20their%20DNA
5. *Risk factors for cancer*. Retrieved April 2025, from https://www.cancer.gov/about-cancer/causes-prevention/risk#:~:text=It%20is%20usually%20not%20possible,factors%2C%20or%20just%20protective%20factors

6. Aghiorghiesei, O., Zanoaga, O., Nutu, A., Braicu, C., Campian, R. S., Lucaciu, O., & Berindan Neagoe, I. (2022). The world of oral cancer and its risk factors viewed from the aspect of MicroRNA expression patterns. *Genes, 13*(4), 594.
7. Hu, J., Dong, H., Dong, Y., Zhou, R., Teixeira, W., He, X., et al. (2024). Cancer burden attributable to risk factors, 1990–2019: A comparative risk assessment. *Iscience, 27*(4), 109430.
8. Irani, S. (2020). New insights into oral cancer—Risk factors and prevention: A review of literature. *International Journal of Preventive Medicine, 11*(1), 202.
9. *Cancer classification*. Retrieved April 2025, from https://training.seer.cancer.gov/disease/categories/classification.html#:~:text=Cancer%20Classification
10. *How is cancer diagnosed?* Stanford Medicine Healthcare
11. Goyal, L., Hingmire, S., & Parikh, P. M. (2006). Newer diagnostic methods in oncology. *Medical Journal, Armed Forces India, 62*(2), 162–168. https://doi.org/10.1016/S0377-1237(06)80062-6
12. Fass, L. (2008). Imaging and cancer: A review. *Molecular Oncology, 2*(2), 115–152. https://doi.org/10.1016/j.molonc.2008.04.001
13. Kaniyala Melanthota, S., et al. (2022). Types of spectroscopy and microscopy techniques for cancer diagnosis: A review. *Lasers in Medical Science, 37*(8), 3067–3084. https://doi.org/10.1007/s10103-022-03610-3
14. Liang, J., Jiang, Y., Abboud, Y., & Gaddam, S. (2022). Role of endoscopy in management of upper gastrointestinal cancers. *Diseases, 11*(1), 3. https://doi.org/10.3390/diseases11010003
15. Teh, J.-L., Shabbir, A., Yuen, S., & So, J. B.-Y. (2020). Recent advances in diagnostic upper endoscopy. *World Journal of Gastroenterology, 26*(4), 433–447. https://doi.org/10.3748/wjg.v26.i4.433
16. *Mouth anatomy*. Retrieved April 2025, from https://emedicine.medscape.com/article/1899122-overview#:~:text=glands%20are%20in%20close%20relation,part%20of%20the%20oral%20cavity
17. Sudhakar, A. (2009). History of cancer, ancient and modern treatment methods. *Journal of Cancer Science and Therapy, 1*(2), i–iv.
18. Hejmadi, M. (2014). *Introduction to cancer biology*. Bookboon.
19. Murthy, N. S., & Mathew, A. (2004). Cancer epidemiology, prevention and control. *Current Science, 86*(4), 518–527.
20. Nagai, H., & Kim, Y. H. (2017). Cancer prevention from the perspective of global cancer burden patterns. *Journal of Thoracic Disease, 9*(3), 448–451.
21. Fitzmaurice, C., Allen, C., Barber, R. M., Barregard, L., Bhutta, Z. A., Brenner, H., et al. (2017). Global, regional, and national cancer incidence, mortality, years of life lost, years lived with disability, and disability-adjusted life-years for 32 cancer groups, 1990 to 2015. *JAMA Oncology, 3*(4), 524.
22. Rivera, C., & Venegas, B. (2014). Histological and molecular aspects of oral squamous cell carcinoma. *Oncology Letters, 8*(1), 7–11.
23. Montero, P. H., & Patel, S. G. (2015). Cancer of the oral cavity. *Surgical Oncology Clinics of North America, 24*(3), 491–508.
24. Dangore–Khasbage, S. (2015). Local metastasis in head and neck cancer—An overview. In L. G. Marcu (Ed.), *Contemporary issues in head and neck cancer management*. IntechOpen.
25. Rao, S. V. K., Mejia, G., Roberts-Thomson, K., & Logan, R. (2013). Epidemiology of oral cancer in Asia in the past decade—An update (2000–2012). *Asian Pacific Journal of Cancer Prevention, 14*(10), 5567–5577.
26. Fan, K. M., Rimal, J., Zhang, P., & Johnson, N. W. (2022). Stark differences in cancer epidemiological data between GLOBOCAN and GBD: Emphasis on oral cancer and wider implications. *eClinicalMedicine, 54*, 101673.
27. Bray, F., Laversanne, M., Sung, H., Ferlay, J., Siegel, R. L., Soerjomataram, I., et al. (2024). Global cancer statistics 2022: GLOBOCAN estimates of incidence and mortality worldwide for 36 cancers in 185 countries. *CA: A Cancer Journal for Clinicians, 74*(3), 229–263.

28. *International agency for research on cancer*. Retrieved April 2025, from https://gco.iarc.fr/today/en
29. Kshersagar, J., Bedge, P., Jagdale, R., Toro, Y., Sharma, S., & Joshi, M. (2020). A review on current scenario of oral cancer in India with special emphasis on modern detection systems and biomarkers. *International Journal of Applied Pharmaceutics, 12*(4), 1–10.
30. ICMR NCDIR. (2020). *Report of National Cancer Registry Programme, 2020 A scientific way to understand about Cancer The Report of National Cancer Registry Programme, 2020 was released on 18*. https://ncdirindia.org
31. Sung, H., Ferlay, J., Siegel, R. L., Laversanne, M., Soerjomataram, I., Jemal, A., et al. (2021). Global cancer statistics 2020: GLOBOCAN estimates of incidence and mortality worldwide for 36 cancers in 185 countries. *CA: A Cancer Journal for Clinicians, 71*(3), 209–249.
32. *Profile of cancer and related factors: Gujarat*. (2021). Bengaluru. https://ncdirindia.org/All_Reports/State_Factsheet_21/Factsheet/FS_Gujarat.pdf
33. Almangush, A., Mäkitie, A. A., Triantafyllou, A., de Bree, R., Strojan, P., Rinaldo, A., et al. (2020). Staging and grading of oral squamous cell carcinoma: An update. *Oral Oncology, 107*, 104799.
34. Patel, A., Gupta, V., Pandya, M., & Shah, S. (2021). Metabolomic profiling of an indian oral squamous cell carcinoma subset. *Analytical Chemistry Letters, 11*(4), 596–606.
35. Bhavika, T., Amisha, P., & Sejal, S. (2018). Human papillomavirus associated burden of oral squamous cell carcinoma in an Indian inhabitants. *Indian Journal of Cancer, 7*(1), 81–100.
36. Muthukrishnan, A., & Warnakulasuriya, S. (2018). Oral health consequences of smokeless tobacco use. *The Indian Journal of Medical Research, 148*(1), 35.
37. Talhout, R., Schulz, T., Florek, E., Van Benthem, J., Wester, P., & Opperhuizen, A. (2011). Hazardous compounds in tobacco smoke. *International Journal of Environmental Research and Public Health, 8*(2), 613–628.
38. Konstantinou, E., Fotopoulou, F., Drosos, A., Dimakopoulou, N., Zagoriti, Z., Niarchos, A., et al. (2018). Tobacco-specific nitrosamines: A literature review. *Food and Chemical Toxicology, 118*, 198–203.
39. Ray, C., Singh, P., Gupta, P., & Sinha, D. (2011). Smokeless tobacco: A major public health problem in the SEA region: A review. *Indian Journal of Public Health, 55*(3), 199.
40. Ram, H., Sarkar, J., Kumar, H., Konwar, R., Bhatt, M. L. B., & Mohammad, S. (2011). Oral cancer: Risk factors and molecular pathogenesis. *Journal of Oral and Maxillofacial Surgery, 10*(2), 132–137.
41. Bano, R., Ahmad, N., Mahagaonkar, A. M., & Latti, R. G. (2011). Study of lung functions in smokers and non-smokers in rural India. *Indian Journal of Physiology and Pharmacology, 55*(1), 84–88.
42. Joshi, P., Dutta, S., Chaturvedi, P., & Nair, S. (2014). Head and neck cancers in developing countries. *Rambam Maimonides Medical Journal, 5*(2), e0009.
43. Saleem, S., Abbasi, Z. A., Hameed, A., Qureshi, N. R., Khan, M. A., & Azhar, A. (2014). Novel p53 codon 240 Ser > Thr coding region mutation in the patients of oral squamous cell carcinoma (OSCC). *Tumour Biology, 35*(8), 7945–7950.
44. Sankaranarayanan, R., Ramadas, K., Amarasinghe, H., Subramanian, S., & Johnson, N. (2015). Oral cancer: Prevention, early detection, and treatment. In H. Gelband, P. Jha, R. Sankaranarayanan, & S. Horton (Eds.), *Cancer: Disease control priorities* (Vol. 3, 3rd ed.). The International Bank for Reconstruction and Development/The World Bank.
45. Sawhney, M., Rohatgi, N., Kaur, J., Shishodia, S., Sethi, G., Gupta, S. D., et al. (2007). Expression of NF-kappaB parallels COX-2 expression in oral precancer and cancer: Association with smokeless tobacco. *International Journal of Cancer, 120*(12), 2545–2556.
46. Macha, M. A., Matta, A., Chauhan, S. S., Siu, K. W. M., & Ralhan, R. (2011). Guggulsterone (GS) inhibits smokeless tobacco and nicotine-induced NF-B and STAT3 pathways in head and neck cancer cells. *Carcinogenesis, 32*(3), 368–380.
47. Saraf, S., Welding, K., Iacobelli, M., Cohen, J. E., Gupta, P. C., & Smith, K. C. (2021). Health warning label compliance for smokeless tobacco products and bidis in five indian states. *Asian Pacific Journal of Cancer Prevention, 22*(S2), 59–64.

48. Sankaran, S., Hiilamo, H., & Glantz, S. A. (2015). Implementation of graphic health warning labels on tobacco products in India: The interplay between the cigarette and the bidi industries. *Tobacco Control, 24*(6), 547–555.
49. McCoy, G. D. (1978). A biochemical approach to the etiology of alcohol related cancers of the head and neck. *Laryngoscope, 88*(1 Pt 2 Suppl 8), 59–62.
50. Wynder, E. L., Bross, E. J., & Feldman, R. M. (1957). A study of the etiological factors in cancer of the mouth. *Cancer, 10*, 1300–1323.
51. O'Grady, I., Anderson, A., & O'Sullivan, J. (2020). The interplay of the oral microbiome and alcohol consumption in oral squamous cell carcinomas. *Oral Oncology, 110*, 105011.
52. Evstifeeva, T. V., & Zaridze, D. G. (1992). Nass use, cigarette smoking, alcohol consumption and risk of oral and oesophageal precancer. *European Journal of Cancer Part B: Oral Oncology, 28*(1), 29–35.
53. Sejal, S. (2016). *Association of genetic alterations of the PI3K AKT pathway with oral squamous cell carcinoma in an Indian subset*. Vallabh Vidyanagar.
54. Ha, P. K., & Califano, J. A. (2004). The role of human papillomavirus in oral carcinogenesis. *Critical Reviews in Oral Biology and Medicine, 15*(4), 188–196.
55. Pal, A., & Kundu, R. (2019). Human papillomavirus E6 and E7: The cervical cancer hallmarks and targets for therapy. *Frontiers in Microbiology, 10*, 3116.
56. Johnson, D. E., Burtness, B., Leemans, C. R., Lui, V. W. Y., Bauman, J. E., & Grandis, J. R. (2020). Head and neck squamous cell carcinoma. *Nature Reviews. Disease Primers, 6*(1), 92.
57. Yete, S., D'Souza, W., & Saranath, D. (2018). High-risk human papillomavirus in oral cancer: Clinical implications. *Oncology, 94*(3), 133–141.
58. Kreimer, A. R., Clifford, G. M., Boyle, P., & Franceschi, S. (2005). Human papillomavirus types in head and neck squamous cell carcinomas worldwide: A systemic review. *Cancer Epidemiology, Biomarkers & Prevention, 14*(2), 467–475.
59. Saberian, E., Jenča, A., Petrášová, A., Jenčová, J., Jahromi, R. A., & Seiffadini, R. (2023). Oral cancer at a glance. *Asian Pacific Journal of Cancer Biology, 8*(4), 379–386.

Chapter 2
Types, Diagnosis, and Treatment of Oral Cancer

Oral cancer encompasses malignancies of the mouth, including the lips, tongue, floor of mouth, cheeks, gums, and palate. This chapter explores the classification of oral cancers by stage and type, methods for early detection and diagnosis, and the various treatment modalities available. Early detection of oral cancer is critical, as the prognosis is significantly better when the cancer is caught at an early stage, for example, localized lip cancers have a 5-year survival rate of about 94%, whereas cancers that have spread distantly have around a 38% survival rate [1]. Below we detail the stages of oral cancer, the common types of tumors, how oral cancer is detected and diagnosed, and the main treatment approaches.

2.1 Stages of Oral Cancer

Cancer staging describes the extent of the disease in the body and is crucial for guiding treatment and estimating prognosis [2, 3]. Oral cancer is often staged using the American Joint Committee on Cancer (AJCC) TNM system, which considers the size/extent of the primary tumor (T), involvement of lymph nodes (N), and presence of distant metastasis (M) [3]. These factors are combined to assign an overall stage from 0 through IV, with a higher stage indicating more advanced disease [3].

While the American Joint Committee on Cancer (AJCC) released its first staging guide in 1977, the International Union Against Cancer (UICC) originally recognized the first version of the TNM staging in 1968 [4]. In 2017, the eighth edition of the UICC and AJCC staging manual (AJCC 8) was released [5]. The details of TNM classification (eighth edition) as per follows:

- **Primary Tumor (T)**
  - **Tx**: Tumor cannot be assessed

R. Thanki, S. Shah, *Artificial Intelligence for Early Detection and Diagnosis of Oral Cancer*, Signals and Communication Technology,
https://doi.org/10.1007/978-3-032-05056-4_2

- **Tis**: Carcinoma in situ
- **T1**: Tumor ≤2 cm and DOI ≤ 5 mm
- **T2**: Tumor ≤2 cm, DOI > 5 mm, and ≤10 mm or tumor >2 cm and ≤4 cm and DOI ≤ 10 mm
- **T3**: Tumor >4 cm or any tumor with DOI > 10 mm
- **T4**: Moderately advanced or very advanced local disease
- **T4a**: Moderately advanced local disease. Tumor invades adjacent structures only (e.g., through cortical bone of mandible or maxilla, or involves the maxillary sinus or skin of the face)
- **T4b**: Very advanced local disease. Tumor invades masticator space, pterygoid plates, or skull base and/or encases the internal carotid artery

• **Nodal Status (N)**

- **Nx**: Regional lymph nodes cannot be assessed
- **N0**: No regional lymph node metastasis
- **N1**: Metastasis in a single ipsilateral lymph node, ≤3 cm and ENE−
- **N2:** Metastasis in a single ipsilateral lymph node >3 cm and ≤6 cm and ENE−; or metastases in multiple ipsilateral lymph nodes, ≤6 cm and ENE−; or in bilateral or contralateral lymph nodes, ≤6 cm and ENE−
- **N2a**: Metastasis in a single ipsilateral lymph node >3 cm and ≤6 cm and ENE
- **N2b:** Metastases in multiple ipsilateral lymph nodes, ≤6 cm and ENE−
- **N2c:** Metastases in bilateral or contralateral lymph nodes, ≤6 cm and ENE−
- **N3:** Metastasis in a lymph node >6 cm and ENE−; or metastasis in any lymph node(s) with ENE+ clinically
- **N3a:** Metastasis in a lymph node >6 cm and ENE−
- **N3b:** Metastasis in any lymph node(s) with ENE+ clinically

• **Metastases (M)**

- **Mx:** Distinct metastasis cannot be accessed
- **M0:** No metastases
- **M1:** Distant metastases present

Tumor grading is being referred to as "stage grouping" and is frequently carried out based on TNM stage (WHO) (as shown in Table 2.1) [3].

Table 2.1 The eighth edition clinical TNM classification of cancer patients

Stage	T	N	M
Stage 0	Tis	N0	M0
Stage I	T1, T2	N0, N1	M0
Stage II	T1, T2	N2	M0
Stage III	T3	N0, N1, N2	
	T4	Any N	M0
	Any T	N3	M0
Stage IV	Any T	Any N	M1

This grading system is based originally by Broder's classification [6], which includes a subjective assessment of mitotic activity, degree of keratinization, and cellular and nuclear pleomorphism. As the cancer progresses, the cell will eventually cease differentiating means that a differentiated cancer cell will resemble a normal cell more, whereas undifferentiated cells will signal an advanced stage of cancer. The cancer is divided into one of the following phases based on its degree of differentiation:

- GX: Impossible to evaluate the grade of differentiation
- G1: Well-differentiated cells have less than 75% keratinization
- G2 (Moderately differentiated): Keratinization ranges from 25% to 75%
- G3: Keratinization is greater than 25% in poorly differentiated
- G4 (Undifferentiated): It has no distinguishing squamous, glandular, or other characteristics

Figure 2.1 shows the steps involved in the pathogenesis of oral squamous cell carcinoma (OSCC). The progression of these stages includes hyperplasia, dysplasia, in situ carcinoma, localized OSCC, early locally advanced, late locally advanced, and metastasized OSCC [7].

Over time, chromosomes and genes are mutated by alcohol, tobacco, oncogenic viruses, and inflammation. Aggressive cancer and premalignant lesions can result from genetic alterations. Tumor suppressor gene inactivation and oncogene activation or amplification are examples of these genetic alterations. Uncontrolled tumor development results from these oncogenes and tumor suppressor gene mutations, which enable tumor cells to proliferate independently and evade growth-inhibitory cues. Tumor cells can multiply and become immortal due to telomere lengthening. Field cancerization hypothesis demonstrates how premalignant development is caused by genetic disruption in the mucosa (Fig. 2.2) [8].

In general, Stage 0 represents carcinoma in situ (very localized cancer), Stages I–II are early-stage invasive cancers, Stage III is a locally advanced or regionally spread cancer, and Stage IV is an advanced cancer that may have spread to adjacent structures or distant organs [2, 3]. The following subsections summarize each stage [2]:

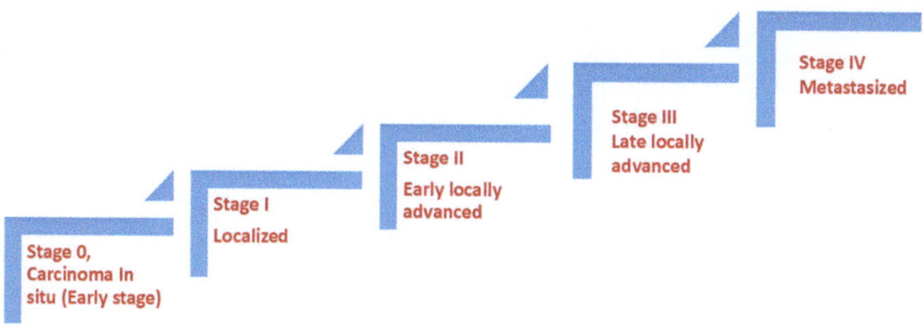

Fig. 2.1 Pathogenesis of OSCC

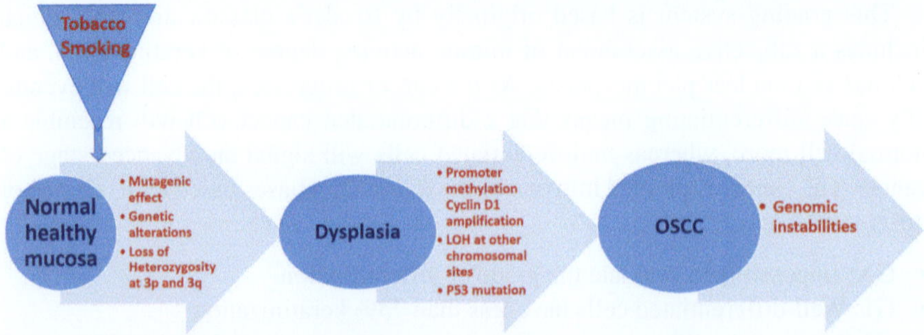

Fig. 2.2 Molecular pathogenesis of OSCC

2.1.1 *Stage 0*

Stage 0 oral cancer is also called carcinoma in situ, in which malignant cells are present only in the most superficial layer of the oral lining and have not invaded deeper tissues [2]. At this stage, the cancer is essentially "pre-invasive." The tumor is confined to the lining epithelium of the mouth or lips and has not spread to any lymph nodes or other organs [2]. Stage 0 lesions are highly curable, often with surgical removal of the abnormal cells, because the disease is caught at its earliest point before any invasion or spread.

2.1.2 *Stage I & II*

Stage I and II oral cancers are considered early-stage invasive cancers. In Stage I, the primary tumor is small, typically 2 cm or less in greatest dimension, with no spread to lymph nodes or distant sites. In Stage II, the tumor is larger than 2 cm but not larger than 4 cm, still without regional lymph node involvement or metastasis. Both Stage I and II tumors are localized to the primary site in the mouth and have not spread, making them potentially curable with definitive local treatment (surgery and/or radiation). These stages differ only by tumor size (Stage II being between 2 and 4 cm). Early-stage oral cancers often present as persistent ulcers or patches in the mouth and may not cause severe symptoms, underscoring the importance of routine oral exams for detection. Prognosis is generally good for Stage I/II cancers, and most patients survive long term when appropriate treatment is given at these stages.

2.1.3 Stage III

Stage III oral cancer indicates a more advanced local disease or initial regional spread. Typically, Stage III is defined in one of two ways: either the primary tumor is larger than 4 cm in size, *or* the cancer has spread to a nearby lymph node (but not distant sites) while the tumor itself may be of smaller/moderate size. For example, a tumor >4 cm with no nodes, or a tumor of any size up to 4 cm that has spread to a single lymph node (on the same side of the neck) no larger than 3 cm, would be classified as Stage III. Stage III thus can represent a sizable, localized tumor or one that has begun regional lymph node involvement. Cancers at this stage often require more aggressive treatment, potentially a combination of surgery and radiation (and sometimes chemotherapy), due to the larger tumor burden or initial nodal spread. The prognosis for Stage III is more guarded than for Stage I/II, but still with a chance for cure, especially if all detectable disease can be removed or eradicated.

2.1.4 Stage IV

Stage IV is the most advanced stage of oral cancer, often subdivided into IVA, IVB, and IVC to indicate specific patterns of spread. In Stage IVA, the tumor may be *any size* but has grown into adjacent tissues such as deeper parts of the tongue, floor of mouth, jawbone (mandible or palate bone), or even the skin of the face or nearby nerves. There may also be spread to regional lymph nodes; typically, in IVA, the lymph nodes contain cancer but are still relatively small (no node larger than 6 cm). Stage IVB often indicates even further local extension (for example, tumor invasion into the base of the skull, involvement of critical structures like the carotid artery, or extensive soft tissue involvement) *or* the presence of large lymph node metastases (a lymph node larger than 6 cm, or cancer in a node that has grown into surrounding tissues). Stage IVC is defined by distant metastasis, the cancer has spread to distant organs such as the lungs, liver, or bones. Any oral cancer with distant metastatic spread is Stage IVC regardless of the primary tumor size. Stage IV oral cancers are often difficult to cure and require multimodal treatment. Patients with Stage IV disease may undergo extensive surgery (to remove the tumor and involved lymph nodes), combined with radiation therapy and chemotherapy or targeted therapies. In cases of very advanced disease (especially Stage IVC), treatment may be palliative, aimed at controlling symptoms and improving quality of life. Overall, the higher the stage, the lower the likelihood of cure; thus, preventing progression to Stage IV through early detection and treatment of oral cancer is a key goal in patient care.

2.2 Types of Oral Cancer

Oral cancers are classified not only by stage but also by their histological type, meaning the kind of cells from which the cancer arises. Most oral cancers are carcinomas—malignancies of epithelial cells that line the mouth. Among these, squamous cell carcinoma (SCC) is by far the most common type, accounting for over 90% of oral malignancies [8]. However, there are several other types of tumors that can occur in the oral cavity, including variants of squamous carcinoma and cancers arising from minor salivary glands, lymphoid tissue, or pigment-producing cells. Below we outline the major types of oral cancer [8]:

2.2.1 *Squamous Cell Carcinoma*

Squamous cell carcinoma is the predominant type of oral cancer. It originates from the squamous cells, the flat, plate-like cells that form the lining (mucosa) of the mouth, tongue, and lips. Chronic exposure to carcinogens like tobacco (smoking or smokeless) and alcohol, as well as human papillomavirus (HPV) infection in some cases, can cause genetic mutations in these cells that lead to SCC. Squamous cell carcinoma of the oral cavity typically appears as a non-healing ulcer, a red or white patch (erythroplakia or leukoplakia that turns cancerous), or an exophytic mass in the mouth. This cancer has the capacity to invade locally into deep tissues and to spread (metastasize) to regional lymph nodes in the neck and, in advanced cases, to distant organs. SCC represents over 90% of all oral and oropharyngeal cancers, making it the focus of most oral cancer prevention and treatment strategies. Depending on the location (tongue, floor of mouth, cheek, etc.), an SCC in the mouth may also be referred to by a specific term (for example, "tongue cancer" is usually squamous carcinoma of the tongue). The prognosis of SCC depends on the stage at diagnosis; early-stage SCC is highly curable with surgery or radiation, whereas advanced SCC can be life-threatening.

2.2.2 *Basal Cell Carcinoma (BCC)*

Basal cell carcinoma is a type of skin cancer that can sometimes affect the lip and perioral region. It arises from the basal cells of the epidermis (the bottom layer of the skin). In the context of oral cancer, basal cell carcinoma is most often discussed in relation to lip cancer. The lips, especially the lower lip, are a transition zone between facial skin and oral mucosa and can develop both squamous cell and basal cell cancers [9, 10]. Basal cell carcinoma of the lip typically occurs on sun-exposed areas (since UV radiation is a major risk factor) and is the second most common type of lip cancer after SCC [10]. It usually presents as a persistent non-healing ulcer or nodule on the lip with a pearly or crusted surface. BCC is characteristically slow growing and *rarely spreads to distant sites*, but it can be locally invasive/destructive if left untreated. Treatment usually involves surgical excision with clear margins. Because basal cell carcinoma is much more common on the skin (like the face) than inside the oral cavity, it is sometimes not classified as an "oral cavity cancer" per se by epidemiologists. However, it's important to recognize it in the lip area. Early detection and removal of lip BCC usually lead to an excellent outcome, given its low metastatic potential.

2.2.3 Oral Verrucous Carcinoma

Verrucous carcinoma is a distinct variant of squamous cell carcinoma that occurs in the oral cavity. It is sometimes called "snuff dipper's cancer" or verrucous *SCC* because it has been linked to smokeless tobacco use. Verrucous carcinoma appears as a slow-growing, warty or cauliflower-like lesion in the mouth often on the gums, cheek, or hard palate. Histologically, it is well-differentiated and tends to push into underlying tissue in a broad, pushing front rather than infiltrating in thin strands. An important feature is that verrucous carcinoma rarely metastasizes (rarely spreads to lymph nodes or distant organs) despite potentially growing quite large locally [8, 9]. It is generally considered a low-grade carcinoma. About 5% of all oral cavity tumors are verrucous carcinomas [9]. Treatment usually involves surgical removal, and prognosis is often good if the entire tumor is excised, though the tumor can be locally aggressive, causing extensive involvement of local tissues if not treated. Sometimes, verrucous carcinoma can transform into a more typical invasive squamous cell carcinoma, so adequate treatment and follow-up are important.

2.2.4 Oral Melanoma, Lymphoma, and Adenoid Cystic Tumors

While carcinomas (like SCC, BCC, and verrucous carcinoma) constitute most oral cancers, other malignant neoplasms can arise in the oral region, though they are relatively rare. These include melanomas, lymphomas, and salivary gland tumors such as adenoid cystic carcinoma [8]:

- **Oral Melanoma:** Malignant melanomas can develop from the pigment-producing cells (melanocytes) in the mucosal lining of the mouth, though this is uncommon. Oral (mucosal) melanoma may appear as a darkly pigmented patch or mass on the gums, palate, or other oral tissues. Between 1% and 2% of all mouth cancers are melanomas, making this a rare subtype [8]. Melanomas in the oral cavity tend to be aggressive and can spread to regional lymph nodes or distant sites. They are treated similarly to melanomas of the skin, often with surgery (wide excision) and sometimes adjuvant immunotherapy. Notably, the behavior and treatment of mucosal melanomas can differ from cutaneous (skin) melanomas, and outcomes are generally poorer due to late detection.

- **Lymphoma:** Cancers of lymphoid tissue can present in the mouth or, more commonly, in the oropharyngeal region. When a lymphoma occurs in oral sites (for example, in the tonsils or base of the tongue, which contain lymphatic tissue), it is not a carcinoma but a malignancy of immune cells (usually B-lymphocytes). Oral lymphomas might manifest as tumors in the tonsil area or extranodal masses in the oral cavity. Oral cancers that develop in lymph tissue such as the tonsils and base of tongue are considered lymphomas [8]. Two common types are non-Hodgkin lymphomas like diffuse large B-cell lymphoma, or Hodgkin lymphoma (rarer in oral location). They are treated primarily with systemic therapy (chemotherapy and/or immunotherapy) rather than surgery, since lymphoma is a systemic disease. The presence of a lymphoma in the oral region can sometimes be mistaken for carcinoma clinically, so biopsy is crucial for correct diagnosis.
- **Adenoid Cystic Carcinoma and Other Salivary Gland Tumors:** The oral cavity and oropharynx have numerous minor salivary glands scattered in the lips, palate, cheek, and throat lining. Malignancies can arise from these glands, although they are infrequent. Adenoid cystic carcinoma (ACC) is an example of a salivary gland cancer that can occur in the oral region. ACC is known for its characteristic cribriform (glandular) microscopic pattern and a tendency for perineural invasion (spreading along nerves). It is an uncommon malignant neoplasm arising from secretory glands, most often the salivary glands of the head and neck [11]. Patients with adenoid cystic carcinoma might notice a firm mass (for instance, on the palate) or experience unexplained pain/numbness due to nerve involvement. ACC typically is slow growing but persistent, and it can recur or metastasize, often to the lungs. Other minor salivary gland cancers include mucoepidermoid carcinoma and polymorphous low-grade adenocarcinoma [8]. Treatment for these salivary cancers usually involves surgery to remove the gland/tumor, often followed by radiation. Long-term follow-up is required, as these tumors can sometimes recur years later.

2.3 Early Detection of Oral Cancer

Early detection of oral cancer significantly improves outcomes. As mentioned, oral cancers caught in initial stages have a much higher survival rate and often can be treated less aggressively than advanced cancers. Unfortunately, many oral cancers are detected at later stages, in part because early lesions can be asymptomatic. Therefore, there is an emphasis on screening examinations and diagnostic techniques to identify oral cancer (or precancerous changes) as early as possible.

Early detection strategies involve two main components: clinical examination (screening) to spot any suspicious lesions, and diagnostic confirmation of those lesions through techniques like biopsy and imaging. Public health campaigns encourage regular dental or medical check-ups that include an oral cancer screening, especially for high-risk individuals (such as tobacco or heavy alcohol users, or those with HPV infection). In this section, we discuss the use of biopsies and imaging in the early detection context.

2.3.1 Biopsies

If an abnormal area is found in the mouth (such as a persistent ulcer, a red or white patch, or an unusual growth), the definitive way to determine whether it is cancerous is to perform a biopsy. A biopsy involves removing a small sample of tissue or cells from the lesion to be examined under a microscope for cancer cells [12]. Biopsy is the gold standard for diagnosing oral cancer, and no screening test or imaging can substitute for the tissue diagnosis. There are different biopsy techniques: an incisional biopsy means cutting out a representative portion of a large lesion, whereas an excisional biopsy means removing the entire lesion (used if the lesion is small). Most oral biopsies can be done under local anesthesia in a clinic setting. For lesions that are difficult to access (e.g., at the base of the tongue or pharynx), the biopsy might be done in an operating room under general anesthesia [13]. In addition to conventional scalpel biopsies, sometimes a fine needle aspiration (FNA) biopsy is used, for instance, to sample cells from an enlarged lymph node in the neck to see if it contains cancer cells [12]. It's worth noting that before doing an invasive biopsy, some practitioners may use adjunctive tests for screening purposes. One example is exfoliative cytology or brush biopsy, where cells are scraped or brushed from the lesion and analyzed (this is less definitive than a tissue biopsy but can indicate if a lesion is suspicious). Ultimately, however, a definitive diagnosis of oral cancer requires a tissue biopsy [12]. Therefore, any persistent oral lesion of unknown cause should be biopsied without undue delay. Early biopsy and diagnosis lead to earlier treatment, which improves the chances of successful outcomes.

2.3.2 Imaging

Imaging techniques play a role in the detection and assessment of oral cancer, though they are often more crucial in staging and planning treatment than in initial screening. In terms of early detection, one aspect of imaging is the use of novel optical devices and techniques to visualize suspicious tissue changes that might not be apparent under normal lighting. For example, tissue autofluorescence imaging devices (like VELscope) have been explored as adjuncts in oral cancer screening. These devices shine a special light in the mouth, causing normal tissue to fluoresce (glow) in a characteristic way; areas of dysplasia or early cancer may appear as dark irregular regions under autofluorescence. Such optical imaging tools are emerging as useful aids in the early diagnosis of oral cancer, helping clinicians spot potentially malignant lesions that warrant biopsy [12]. Another adjunct technique is the application of toluidine blue dye to the oral mucosa, this dye tends to selectively stain abnormal cells, highlighting areas that could be precancerous or cancerous. Studies show toluidine blue has a high sensitivity (it will stain most true cancers) but only moderate specificity (it may also stain some benign changes), making it a helpful guide to choose biopsy sites.

Beyond these specialized tools, traditional imaging modalities are used once an oral lesion is identified, to evaluate the extent of the tumor. For example, a dentist or oral surgeon who finds a suspicious lesion might order a radiograph (X-ray) of the jaws or a CT scan or MRI to see how deep the tumor extends or if bone is involved. While imaging is not used to diagnose oral cancer initially (one cannot confirm cancer on a scan alone without a biopsy), it is used to detect the full extent of a known tumor and to look for hidden spread [12]. Common imaging tests include:

- **CT (Computed Tomography) scans** which provide detailed cross-sectional images and are excellent for detecting tumors in the jaw, palate, or checking for lymph node enlargement and lung metastases. A CT scan can show the tumor's size, any invasion into adjacent tissues, and enlarged lymph nodes [12].
- **MRI (Magnetic Resonance Imaging) scans** which give high-contrast images of soft tissues, useful for tongue and floor of mouth cancers to delineate tumor boundaries in muscle.
- **Ultrasound:** Occasionally used for evaluating neck lymph nodes or guiding needle biopsies.
- **PET scans (Positron Emission Tomography):** Often combined with CT (PET/CT) to detect metabolic activity of cancer and reveal cancer spread that might not be obvious on anatomic imaging, especially in advanced cases.

In summary, imaging in early detection is mainly about adjunctive visualization tools to find lesions (like fluorescence devices) and initial radiographic exams to map out a discovered lesion's extent. The combined use of careful clinical exam (visual inspection and palpation), adjunct screening tools, and prompt biopsy of any suspicious area gives the best chance of catching oral cancer at an early, more treatable stage.

2.4 Diagnosis of Oral Cancer

The diagnosis of oral cancer is a multi-step process that includes screening examinations, definitive diagnostic procedures, and staging workup once a cancer is confirmed. "Diagnosis" in this context covers both identifying that a patient has oral cancer and determining the cancer's exact nature and extent. We will discuss two important aspects: screening (how patients are examined for possible signs of oral cancer) and staging (how, after diagnosis, the cancer is categorized by extent).

2.4.1 Screening

Screening refers to examining people for signs of cancer before symptoms develop. For oral cancer, there is no large-scale population screening program (unlike, say, mammograms for breast cancer) for the general population, partly due to conflicting evidence on whether it reduces mortality [3]. However, opportunistic screening by healthcare professionals (such as dentists, dental hygienists, or primary care physicians) during routine visits is very important, especially in individuals with risk factors.

An oral cancer screening exam is quick and non-invasive. Guidelines for an adequate oral cancer screening indicate that the clinician should take a thorough history (looking for risk factors like tobacco, alcohol use, prior cancer, or HPV status) and perform a systematic examination of all oral and pharyngeal tissues [2, 3]. This includes inspection of the lips, tongue (including lifting the tongue to inspect the floor of mouth and the underside and sides of the tongue), the buccal mucosa (inner cheeks), gums, palate, and back of the throat. Palpation (feeling with fingers) is also crucial, and the examiner will feel for any lumps or indurations in the oral tissues and in the neck (lymph node areas). A piece of gauze might be used to grab and move the tongue for a better view of the base of tongue and throat regions [12]. Good lighting and sometimes special tools like mouth mirrors are needed to visualize all areas.

During screening, the provider looks for early signs of oral cancer or pre-cancer, such as persistent white patches (leukoplakia) or red patches (erythroplakia) that don't rub off, non-healing ulcers, unexplained bleeding, swelling or thickening of tissues, or any asymmetry/mass. They also check cranial nerve function (for example, tongue movement and sensation) because nerve involvement can indicate deeper tumor invasion [12].

If any suspicious area is found, the practitioner will typically recommend a diagnostic workup (as described in Sect. 2.3, usually a biopsy). Patient education is also a part of screening—people are advised to report any mouth sore that doesn't heal within 2 weeks, any unexplained pain, or difficulty swallowing. High-risk individuals (heavy smokers and drinkers) should ideally have an annual oral exam. Some dental clinics offer adjunctive screening tools like toluidine blue rinses or autofluorescence lights as part of the exam, although these are supplementary.

It's important to note that while screening exams are valuable, they are not foolproof. Some early cancers may be hard to distinguish from benign conditions. Nonetheless, screening is our best tool for early detection: it's simple, low-cost, and can be lifesaving if it finds an oral cancer before it progresses. On the public health side, efforts to raise awareness (for example, oral cancer awareness campaigns) aim to encourage both providers and patients to be vigilant. Early diagnosis of oral cancer via screening leads to earlier intervention and a markedly improved prognosis [14].

2.4.2 Staging

Once a diagnosis of oral cancer is confirmed by biopsy, the staging process begins. Staging was introduced earlier (Sect. 2.1) in terms of what the stages mean. Here we focus on *how* staging is done in practice as part of the diagnostic evaluation. Staging determines how extensive the cancer is including the size of the primary tumor and whether it has spread to lymph nodes or other organs. Proper staging is essential for formulating an optimal treatment plan and for predicting the patient's prognosis [2].

The most used staging scheme for oral cancer is the TNM system developed by the AJCC/UICC (was described earlier in Sect. 2.1). As noted, *T* (tumor) is assessed by measuring the tumor and seeing how far it invades locally; *N* (nodes) is assessed by examining and imaging the regional lymph nodes of the neck for cancer spread; *M* (metastasis) is assessed by looking for cancer in distant sites like the lungs, liver, etc. [4, 5]. Each letter gets a numerical sub-classification (for example, T1, T2, T3, T4 depending on size/extent; N0 means no nodes, N1/N2 etc. depending on number/size of nodes; M0 means no metastasis, M1 means distant metastasis present). These are then combined to yield an overall stage group (I, II, III, IV).

Clinical staging starts with a thorough head and neck examination. The doctor will carefully feel for any enlarged lymph nodes in the neck (since even non-visible metastasis can sometimes be palpable as a firm node). Imaging studies are integral to staging: a CT scan or MRI of the oral region and neck is usually performed to determine the exact tumor size and involvement of adjacent structures [4]. Imaging also helps detect lymph nodes that are suspicious even if not palpable. A chest X-ray or CT scan of the chest is commonly done to check the lungs for any spread (the lungs are a common site of metastasis for oral cancer) [12]. In some cases, a PET-CT scan is done for a more sensitive whole-body survey for metastasis.

Sometimes an examination under anesthesia (EUA) is conducted by the surgeon to palpate and assess the tumor and adjacent areas more thoroughly than might be possible in the clinic. Additional biopsies or procedures might be done during staging, such as a pan endoscopy (scoping the esophagus and airway) to rule out second primaries (patients with oral SCC can have simultaneous cancers elsewhere in the head-neck region or esophagus).

After gathering all this information, the cancer is assigned a TNM stage. For example, a 1.5 cm tongue tumor with no nodes is T1 N0 M0 = Stage I; a 3 cm floor of mouth tumor with one small lymph node metastasis might be T2 N1 M0 = Stage III; a 5 cm tumor invading the jaw with multiple large lymph nodes might be T4a N2 M0 = Stage IVA, and so on. The stage grouping is essentially a summary: early stage (I/II), locally advanced (III/IVA/IVB depending on nodes and invasion), or metastatic (IVC).

Staging not only guides treatment choices (for instance, Stage I might be treated with single-modality surgery or radiation, whereas Stage III or IV often needs multimodal therapy), but also informs prognosis discussions [4, 5]. It's worth emphasizing that the diagnostic stage (called the clinical stage) may sometimes be adjusted if surgery is done pathologists examine the removed tissue and lymph nodes, and occasionally they find more involvement than expected, leading to a pathologic stage that might be higher. However, the clinical stage is what's used to plan initial treatment.

In summary, diagnosing oral cancer involves confirming the malignancy via biopsy and then accurately staging the disease using exams and imaging. The result of the diagnostic phase is a clear understanding of what the cancer is (histological type), where it is, and how far it has spread, so that an appropriate treatment strategy can be formulated.

2.5 Treatment for Oral Cancer

The treatment of oral cancer typically involves one or more of the following modalities: surgery, radiation therapy, chemotherapy, and newer systemic treatments like targeted therapy and immunotherapy. The choice of treatment (or combination of treatments) depends on the cancer's stage, location, and type, as well as the patient's overall health and personal preferences. Early-stage oral cancers might be cured with a single treatment (surgery or radiation), whereas advanced stages often require a combination (for example, surgery followed by radiation and chemotherapy). Below we discuss each of the main treatment approaches [15]:

2.5.1 Surgery

Surgical removal of the cancer is a cornerstone of treatment for most oral cancers, especially those that are localized (Stages I–III). Surgery involves excising the tumor along with a margin of normal tissue to ensure clear boundaries, this is to reduce the risk of leaving behind microscopic cancer cells. For example, a small tumor on the tongue can be removed via partial glossectomy (removal of part of the tongue) with a margin of healthy tissue. If the cancer has invaded the jawbone or other structures, the surgeon will remove those involved portions (such as performing a mandibulectomy for jaw involvement) [15]. The extent of surgery is determined by the tumor's size and spread: "The extent of the surgery depends on the size of the cancer. If cancer has spread into bone, the surgeon may remove some bone tissue" [15].

In addition to removing the primary tumor, oral cancer surgery often includes addressing the regional lymph nodes. Many patients undergo a neck dissection, which is a surgery to remove lymph nodes in the neck that might harbor cancer cells [15]. Even if lymph nodes are not obviously involved (clinically N0), surgeons may remove at least a few nodes as a precaution in cases where there's significant risk of microscopic spread [15]. Removing and examining lymph nodes also provide accurate staging (was there hidden spread?) and can guide the need for additional therapy.

One of the challenges of oral cancer surgery is that removing tumors in the mouth can affect appearance and function (speech, chewing, swallowing). Therefore, surgical planning often includes considerations for reconstruction. Reconstructive surgery may be done during the same operation if large amounts of tissue are removed, for instance, grafting skin, muscle, or bone from another part of the body to rebuild the tongue or jaw (this is known as flap reconstruction) [15]. Rehabilitation (such as speech therapy and swallowing therapy) is often needed after major oral surgeries [15].

Surgery offers the advantage of physically removing the cancer in one go. For early-stage cancers, surgery alone can often be curative. In more advanced cases, surgery is usually combined with other treatments (e.g., postoperative radiation or chemoradiation) to kill any residual cancer cells. Surgical risk includes typical risks of anesthesia and operations (bleeding, infection) and the specific risks like changes in the ability to speak or eat [15]. Still, with modern techniques and reconstructive options, many patients can return to a good quality of life after recovering from oral cancer surgery.

2.5.2 Chemotherapy

Chemotherapy uses anti-cancer drugs to destroy cancer cells throughout the body. In oral cancer management, chemotherapy is often used as an adjunct to other treatments rather than the sole treatment. The most common scenario is using chemotherapy in combination with radiation therapy, a strategy known as chemoradiation. Certain drugs (like cisplatin) make cancer cells more sensitive to radiation, thereby increasing the effectiveness of the radiation in killing the tumor. "Chemotherapy may increase the effectiveness of radiation therapy, so the two treatments are often combined." [15]. This combined approach is frequently employed in advanced stage III or IV cancers, especially if the goal is to avoid surgery or to treat residual disease after surgery [15].

Chemotherapy for oral cancer typically involves agents such as cisplatin, 5-fluorouracil (5-FU), carboplatin, or in some cases taxanes (like docetaxel). These may be given singly or in combination. For example, in a stage IV oral cancer, a patient might receive cisplatin concurrent with radiation as part of definitive organ-preserving therapy, or post-operatively if there were high-risk features in surgery.

Chemotherapy is also used in palliative settings—if oral cancer has spread to distant organs and is not curable by surgery or radiation, chemotherapy can help shrink tumors and alleviate symptoms, prolonging survival (though it is not curative in that scenario) [15]. In recent years, chemotherapy might also be combined with newer targeted drugs or immunotherapy for recurrent/metastatic oral cancers.

Like all systemic treatments, chemo can cause side effects. Common side effects include nausea, vomiting, hair loss, fatigue, oral ulcers, and increased risk of infection due to lowered blood counts. These side effects depend on the specific drugs and doses used. The oncology team will manage side effects with supportive medications (like anti-nausea drugs) and dose adjustments as needed.

In summary, chemotherapy plays a supportive yet important role in oral cancer treatment. It is often used after surgery (adjuvant therapy) to eliminate microscopic disease [15], or concurrently with radiation to enhance tumor kill. For later-stage disease, it can help control the cancer's spread. The integration of chemotherapy into a treatment plan is usually determined by the cancer's stage and pathological features. For instance, multiple positive lymph nodes or extracapsular spread in nodes usually warrant adding chemoradiation after surgery, because studies have shown this approach improves patient outcomes.

2.5.3 Radiation Therapy

Radiation therapy uses high-energy radiation (X-rays or other particles like protons) to destroy cancer cells. In oral cancer, radiation can be delivered externally by a machine that rotates around the head and neck (external beam radiation) or internally via radioactive sources placed near the tumor (brachytherapy). External beam radiation (often using advanced techniques like IMRT (intensity modulated radiation therapy) to precisely target the tumor) is the more common method for oral cancers.

Radiation therapy might be employed in different roles: as a primary treatment for small cancers, as a post-surgery adjuvant treatment, or for palliation. For a very early-stage oral cancer (like a small lip cancer or early tongue cancer in a patient who cannot undergo surgery), radiation alone might be curative. More often, radiation is used after surgical removal of the tumor to kill any remaining cancer cells that are too small to be seen (microscopic residual disease). This is particularly indicated if the tumor had close or positive margins, multiple lymph node involvement, or perineural/vascular invasion. Sometimes chemotherapy is given along with radiation (chemoradiation) because chemo drugs like cisplatin can sensitize cancer cells to radiation and improve the efficacy though this combined approach can also increase side effects. In advanced scenarios where the cancer cannot be completely removed or has spread, radiation can be used to relieve symptoms such as pain, bleeding, or difficulty swallowing by shrinking the tumors (palliative radiation).

Radiation therapy for oral cancer is very effective at killing cancer cells, but it inevitably affects normal tissues in the treatment field. Thus, side effects are an important consideration. Side effects of radiation to the oral region often include dry mouth (xerostomia) due to salivary gland damage, changes in taste, soreness of the mucous membranes (mucositis), dental problems and tooth decay (radiation can harm teeth and jawbone blood supply), and risk of osteoradionecrosis (bone damage) in the jaw. Patients are usually advised to see a dentist prior to radiation to address any dental issues and possibly remove high-risk teeth, because radiation can impair healing. During radiation, meticulous oral hygiene, and certain protective agents can help mitigate side effects.

A special form of radiation, brachytherapy, involves placing radioactive sources directly in the tumor area (for instance, needles or catheters in a tumor bed in the tongue or lip). This is less commonly used than external beam for oral cancer, but can be an option for some cases, either alone (for very small, accessible tumors) or in combination with external radiation.

Overall, radiation therapy is a critical modality in oral cancer care. It is often part of combined treatment plans and has the advantage of preserving structures (for example, organ-preservation in oropharyngeal cancers with chemoradiation as an alternative to radical surgery). The decision to use radiation, and the scheduling relative to surgery or chemo, is made by a multidisciplinary team considering the tumor's characteristics.

2.5.4 Targeted Therapy

Targeted therapy refers to medications that specifically target molecular features of cancer cells, for example, a protein or pathway that the cancer cells rely on to inhibit cancer growth with potentially fewer side effects than traditional chemotherapy. In oral cancers (most of which are squamous cell carcinomas of the head and neck), the most well-known targeted therapy is a class of drugs that target the Epidermal Growth Factor Receptor (EGFR). EGFR is often overexpressed in head and neck squamous cell carcinomas, helping the cancer cells grow and divide.

A prime example of a targeted drug in oral cancer is cetuximab (Erbitux), a monoclonal antibody that binds to EGFR on cancer cells. By blocking EGFR, cetuximab can slow or stop the growth of the cancer cells [16]. Cetuximab is an FDA-approved targeted therapy for certain head and neck cancers. It can be used in combination with radiation for locally advanced cancers or with chemotherapy for more advanced cases [16]. For instance, a patient who cannot tolerate the side effects of standard chemotherapy might receive cetuximab with radiation as an alternative regimen in a locally advanced oral cancer [16].

Targeted therapy may be given alone or with other treatments. In recurrent or metastatic oral cancer, cetuximab can be combined with chemo (a regimen known as the "EXTREME" regimen: platinum +5-FU + cetuximab) to improve survival. In some cases of less advanced disease, cetuximab with radiation has shown effectiveness.

The side effect profile of targeted therapies differs from general chemo. For EGFR inhibitors like cetuximab, common side effects include an acne-like rash, itching, fatigue, and potentially infusion reactions (allergic-like reactions when the drug is given intravenously). Interestingly, because EGFR is also involved in skin and hair follicles, patients often get skin issues, and sun-sensitivity is a known effect (patients are advised to use sun protection) [16]. It's important to note that targeted therapies are chosen based on the presence of the target. EGFR is ubiquitous enough in head/neck SCC that cetuximab can be broadly applied. Future targets may include specific genetic mutations or pathways, but as of the mid-2020s, cetuximab is the main targeted drug widely in use for oral cavity cancers.

Research is ongoing to develop and validate other targeted treatments. Some oral cancers might have mutations (like in PIK3CA, etc.) that can be targeted by experimental drugs in clinical trials. But as far as standard care goes, monoclonal antibody therapy against EGFR is the hallmark targeted approach for head and neck/oral cancers [16].

2.5.5 Immunotherapy

Immunotherapy is a newer pillar of cancer treatment that helps the patient's own immune system recognize and fight cancer cells. Certain oral cancers, especially those that are advanced or have recurred after initial treatments, can be treated with immunotherapy drugs known as immune checkpoint inhibitors. These drugs "take the brakes off" the immune cells so they can attack the cancer.

The two main immunotherapy agents used in oral (and more broadly, head and neck) cancers are pembrolizumab (Keytruda) and nivolumab (Opdivo). These are monoclonal antibodies that target a checkpoint protein called PD-1 on T-cells [17]. Normally, PD-1 acts as a switch to dampen immune responses (preventing autoimmunity). Tumor cells often exploit this by expressing PD-1's ligands (PDL1) to turn off T-cells. By blocking PD-1, drugs like pembrolizumab and nivolumab release the inhibition on T-cells, allowing the immune system to better recognize and destroy cancer cells [17].

For oral cavity cancers, immunotherapy is generally used in advanced settings specifically, when the cancer is recurrent (has come back after prior treatment) or metastatic (stage IVC), and is not responding to conventional therapies [17]. Pembrolizumab or nivolumab can shrink tumors or slow their growth in a subset of patients, significantly prolonging survival in some cases. In fact, pembrolizumab is now an approved first-line treatment (sometimes given with chemotherapy) for metastatic or unresectable recurrent head and neck squamous carcinomas that express PD-L1, as it has shown better outcomes compared to chemotherapy alone [17].

Immunotherapy is given as an intravenous infusion, every few weeks. One advantage is that it tends to be better tolerated than traditional chemotherapy for many patients. However, immunotherapy can cause unique side effects known as immune-related adverse events, where the activated immune system may attack normal organs. Common side effects include fatigue, rash, and diarrhea, but more serious ones can involve the lungs (pneumonitis), liver (hepatitis), endocrine glands (thyroid or pituitary dysfunction), etc. [17]. These side effects are relatively infrequent and often manageable with steroids or other immunosuppressants if caught early. Many patients do not experience severe issues and can stay on immunotherapy for extended periods if the cancer is responding.

To summarize, immunotherapy has added an important option for oral cancer treatment, especially in advanced cases that have limited options. By harnessing the immune system, these therapies have achieved durable responses in some patients who previously had very poor prognoses. As research progresses, there is hope that immunotherapy could be moved earlier in treatment or combined with other therapies to further improve outcomes for oral cancer patients.

Modern treatment of oral cancer is multidisciplinary. Early-stage cancers are often cured with single-modality therapy (surgery or radiation). Locally advanced cancers typically require combination therapy (surgery plus postoperative chemoradiation or definitive chemoradiation) to achieve control. Recurrent or metastatic cancers may be managed with systemic therapies like chemotherapy, targeted agents, or immunotherapy to prolong life and relieve symptoms. The treatment plan should be individualized, ideally discussed by a tumor board (a team of surgeons, oncologists, radiologists, etc.), to coordinate the best approach for the patient. Through advances in surgery, reconstruction, radiation technology, and drug therapies, the outlook for oral cancer continues to improve, especially when it is detected and treated promptly [17]. Each modality comes with its benefits and risks, and patients often receive a combination tailored to maximize tumor control while maintaining quality of life.

References

1. *Survival rates for oral cavity and oropharyngeal cancer*. Retrieved April 2025, from https://www.cancer.org/cancer/types/oral-cavity-and-oropharyngeal-cancer/detection-diagnosis-staging/survival-rates.html#:~:text=Localized
2. *Stages of oral cancer*. Retrieved April 2025, from https://cancer.ca/en/cancer-information/cancer-types/oral/staging#:~:text=Staging%20describes%20or%20classifies%20a,your%20prognosis
3. *Oral cavity and oropharyngeal cancer stages*. Retrieved April 2025, from https://www.cancer.org/cancer/types/oral-cavity-and-oropharyngeal-cancer/detection-diagnosis-staging/staging.html#:~:text=The%20earliest%20stage%20oral%20cavity,in%20much%20the%20same%20way
4. Almangush, A., Mäkitie, A. A., Triantafyllou, A., de Bree, R., Strojan, P., Rinaldo, A., et al. (2020). Staging and grading of oral squamous cell carcinoma: an update. *Oral Oncology, 107*, 104799.
5. Amin, M. B., Edge, S. B., Greene, F. L., Byrd, D. R., Brookland, R. K., Washington, M. K., et al. (2017). *AJCC cancer staging manual* (Vol. 1024). Springer.
6. Broders, A. C. (1941). The microscopic grading of cancer. *The Surgical Clinics of North America, 21*, 947–962.
7. Hunter, K. D., Parkinson, E. K., & Harrison, P. R. (2005). Profiling early head and neck cancer. *Nature Reviews Cancer, 5*(2), 127–135.
8. *Types of mouth and oropharyngeal cancers*. Retrieved May 2025, from https://www.cancerresearchuk.org/about-cancer/mouth-cancer/stages-types-grades/types-grades#:~:text=throat
9. *Oral cancer types*. Retrieved May 2025, from https://www.cancercenter.com/cancer-types/oral-cancer/types#:~:text=Lip%20cancer
10. *Lip cancer*. Retrieved May 2025, from https://www.hopkinsmedicine.org/health/conditions-and-diseases/lip-cancer#:~:text=The%20second,it%20can%20be%20locally%20aggressive

11. *Adenoid cystic carcinoma*. Retrieved May 2025, from https://oralcancerfoundation.org/facts/rare/adenoid-cystic-carcinoma/#:~:text=Adenoid%20cystic%20carcinoma%20,by%20its%20distinctive%20histologic%20appearance
12. *Tests for oral cavity and oropharyngeal cancers*. Retrieved May 2025, from https://www.cancer.org/cancer/types/oral-cavity-and-oropharyngeal-cancer/detection-diagnosis-staging/how-diagnosed.html#:~:text=Biopsy
13. *Early detection, diagnosis and staging*. Retrieved May 2025, from https://oralcancerfoundation.org/cdc/early-detection-diagnosis-staging/#:~:text=match%20at%20L252%20A%20definitive,of%20the%20lesion%2C%20with%20a
14. Morikawa, T., Shibahara, T., Nomura, T., Katakura, A., & Takano, M. (2020). Non-invasive early detection of oral cancers using fluorescence visualization with optical instruments. *Cancer, 12*(10), 2771.
15. *Mouth cancer*. Retrieved May 2025, from https://www.mayoclinic.org/diseases-conditions/mouth-cancer/diagnosis-treatment/drc-20351002#:~:text=During%20mouth%20cancer%20surgery%2C%20the,the%20margin%20helps%20ensure%20that
16. *Targeted therapy for oral cavity and oropharyngeal cancer*. Retrieved May 2025, from https://www.cancer.org/cancer/types/oral-cavity-and-oropharyngeal-cancer/treating/targeted-therapy.html#:~:text=EGFR,or%20stop%20cancer%20cell%20growth
17. *Immunotherapy for oral cavity and oropharyngeal cancer*. Retrieved May 2025, from https://www.cancer.org/cancer/types/oral-cavity-and-oropharyngeal-cancer/treating/immunotherapy.html#:~:text=Pembrolizumab%20,tumors%20or%20slow%20their%20growth

Chapter 3
Artificial Intelligence and Its Role in Early Detection of Oral Cancer

Oral cancer, predominantly manifesting as oral squamous cell carcinoma (OSCC), represents a significant and escalating global health challenge. It ranks as the sixth most common cancer worldwide, contributing to substantial morbidity and mortality, particularly when diagnoses are rendered at advanced stages [1]. The prognosis for oral cancer is intrinsically linked to the stage at detection; prompt diagnosis coupled with appropriate management can yield a 5-year relative survival rate approaching 90% [1]. Conversely, a diagnosis at a later, more advanced stage dramatically curtails these survival prospects [1]. This stark contrast underscores an urgent and critical imperative for innovative and effective strategies aimed at facilitating early detection.

The ramifications of late-stage oral cancer detection extend beyond individual patient outcomes, imposing a considerable socioeconomic burden. This is especially pronounced in regions with high incidence rates, such as India, where oral cancer is a leading malignancy [1]. The complexity and cost associated with managing advanced disease contribute significantly to healthcare expenditures and loss of productive life years [1]. Consequently, the successful implementation of early AI-driven detection methodologies holds the promise not only of improving survival rates but also of alleviating this broader public health and economic strain by reducing the necessity for resource-intensive late-stage interventions.

Artificial intelligence (AI) has emerged as a transformative force within the healthcare sector, heralding a paradigm shift in oncological diagnostics and care [2]. The inherent capacity of AI to meticulously process and analyze vast, complex datasets, discern subtle patterns often imperceptible to human clinicians, and iteratively learn from new information presents unprecedented opportunities [2]. These capabilities are being harnessed to enhance various facets of cancer management, including early detection, diagnostic accuracy, prognostic assessment, and the formulation of personalized treatment strategies [3].

R. Thanki, S. Shah, *Artificial Intelligence for Early Detection and Diagnosis of Oral Cancer*, Signals and Communication Technology,
https://doi.org/10.1007/978-3-032-05056-4_3

A fundamental limitation in traditional diagnostic pathways for oral cancer is the often-unreliable nature of its clinical presentation in predicting disease status, progression, or the degree of dysplasia [1]. This unreliability can precipitate diagnostic delays and inaccuracies, thereby compromising timely and effective intervention. AI, with its objective, data-driven analytical prowess, is uniquely positioned to address this challenge. By moving beyond subjective clinical assessments, AI offers the potential to provide more consistent, accurate, and early diagnostic insight, thereby overcoming a core deficiency in conventional approaches.

This chapter provides an expert-level analysis of the evolving and critical role of AI in the early detection of oral cancer. It will commence with a foundation definition of AI and an exploration of its broader applications within the healthcare landscape and general oncology. Subsequently, the report will delve into specific AI methodologies and their deployment across the various stages' integral to the diagnosis of oral cancer. Drawing upon current research findings, this chapter will also critically provide the attendant with challenges, inherent limitations, and promising further proposed of AI in this specialized domain.

3.1 Artificial Intelligence

3.1.1 Core Concepts and Technologies of AI

Artificial Intelligence (AI) is a comprehensive and rapidly advancing field of science dedicated to the creation of computers and machines endowed with capabilities that traditionally necessitate human intelligence. These capabilities include reasoning, learning, problem-solving, perception, language understanding, and decision-making, often involving datasets whose scale and complexity exceed human analytical capacity [4]. From an operational perspective, particularly in business and practical applications, AI is conceptualized as a suite of technologies. These are predominantly found on machine learning and deep learning paradigms and are employed for a diverse array of functions, such as sophisticated data analytics, predictive modeling and forecasting, object categorization, natural language processing (NLP), personalized recommendation systems, and intelligent data retrieval [4]. The fundamental mechanism by which AI systems operate involves learning from and iteratively improving through exposure to vast quantities of data. By processing this data, AI algorithms identify intricate patterns, correlations, and relationships that might be imperceptible to human observers, with their analysis and decision-making processes guided by predefined algorithms sets of rules or instructions [4].

The evolution of AI from concepts like "Reactive Machines," which operate solely based on preprogrammed rules without the ability to learn from new data (e.g., IBM's Deep Blue) to "Limited Memory" AI, which characterizes most modern AI systems, is a pivotal development for its application in healthcare. Reactive machines would be insufficient for the dynamic and evolving nature of medical tasks. In contrast, limited memory AI can improve its performance over time by being trained with new data, a characteristic that is fundamental for medical applications where knowledge bases and patient data are constantly expanding. This capacity for learning and adaptation is what makes current AI a viable and powerful tool in medicine. Future progress toward more advanced AI stages, such as "Theory of Mind" AI envisioned to emulate human-like understanding of emotions and social contexts could signify further transformative leaps in AI's medical capabilities, potentially enabling more nuanced patient interaction and complex clinical reasoning [4].

3.1.2 Key Subfields: Machine Learning, Deep Learning, and Their Relevance

Machine Learning (ML) stands as a significant subset of AI. In ML, algorithms are not explicitly programmed for each specific task; instead, they are "trained" using large datasets either labeled (supervised learning) or unlabeled (unsupervised learning) to learn patterns and make predictions or categorize new, unseen information [4]. This allows computer systems to learn from historical data, extract valuable insights, and apply these learned models to make informed predictions about future data. Within the oncological domain, supervised ML methodologies, such as Support Vector Machines (SVMs) and Random Forest algorithms, are extensively utilized. These algorithms analyze patterns within existing patient datasets to facilitate tumor classification, predict prognosis, and identify individuals at higher risk [5].

Deep Learning (DL) is a specialized subfield of ML that employs artificial neural networks with multiple layers, hence "deep" neural networks, to learn highly complex patterns and representations from vast and often unstructured datasets [4]. A key advantage of DL methods is their ability to automatically learn relevant features from the data (feature learning) and integrate this into the model-building process. This reduces the reliance on manually engineered features, which can be incomplete or suboptimal, and enables the development of end-to-end prediction models that map raw input data directly to outputs [6].

DL techniques, particularly Convolutional Neural Networks (CNNs), have demonstrated exceptional efficacy in the analysis of medical images, including tasks such as image classification (e.g., identifying cancerous vs. non-cancerous tissue), segmentation (e.g., delineating tumor boundaries), and detection (e.g., locating suspicious lesions) [6]. Another class of DL models, Recurrent Neural Networks (RNNs), are adept at processing sequential data, such as text. In oncology, RNNs are applied in Natural Language Processing (NLP) tasks, for instance, to extract clinically significant information from unstructured pathology reports or electronic health records [5].

The profoundly interdisciplinary nature of AI, drawn from computer science, data analytics, statistics, hardware and software engineering, linguistics, neuroscience, and even philosophy and psychology [5], suggests that significant advancements in AI for healthcare are unlikely to emerge from a single discipline in isolation. Instead, they will likely arise from synergistic collaborations across these diverse fields. Healthcare problems themselves are multifaceted, involving intricate biological, physiological, psychological, and social factors. Consequently, the inherent interdisciplinarity of AI makes it particularly well-suited for addressing these complex healthcare challenges. This, however, underscores the critical need for robust and active collaboration between AI specialists and domain experts, such as medical researchers, clinicians, and pathologists, to ensure that AI solutions are clinically relevant, ethically sound, and effectively integrated into practice. This points toward a broader need for interdisciplinary training programs and research funding models that actively foster such partnerships to fully realize AI's transformative potential in medicine.

3.2 AI in Healthcare Research

3.2.1 Broad Applications of AI in Clinical Medicine

Artificial Intelligence is poised to revolutionize numerous aspects of clinical medicine, primarily through its capacity to manage, interpret, and derive insights from the large and complex datasets routinely generated within healthcare services [2]. The potential applications of AI are extensive, spanning the entire continuum of patient care. This includes enhancing diagnostic processes, improving prognostic accuracy, guiding clinical decision-making, optimizing treatment strategies, facilitating patient education, and supporting follow-up care [2]. AI systems can rapidly process vast quantities of patient data, identify subtle yet significant patterns that might elude human clinicians, and learn from historical diagnostic successes and errors [7]. A notable capability is AI's potential to encompass a comprehensive knowledge base of symptoms and diseases, which can be invaluable in assisting patients who present with ambiguous or rare symptoms that fall between traditional medical specializations [7].

The integration of AI into clinical practice, however, is still in its nascent stages, and a clear, comprehensive quantification of its benefits is an ongoing endeavor [2]. The "dataset ceiling effect" represents a critical and often underappreciated limitation in this context [2]. If AI models are trained exclusively on existing Electronic Health Record (EHR) data, which may contain inherent diagnostic errors or unrecorded misdiagnoses, these models will inevitably learn to replicate these inaccuracies. Consequently, such AI systems might only achieve an accuracy level comparable to the current healthcare system, including its human errors, rather than surpassing it [7]. This implies that AI could, in some instances, learn to reproduce these errors with even greater efficiency. This highlights a fundamental prerequisite for achieving true diagnostic improvement through AI: the development of "gold-standard," meticulously curated, and verified training datasets. This necessity for high-quality data signifies that simply applying AI to readily available EHR data is insufficient. It points toward a significant, resource-intensive effort required to create these specialized datasets, which, while potentially slowing the immediate translation of some AI tools into clinical practice, is crucial for ensuring their ultimate quality, safety, and efficacy.

3.2.2 Potential to Revolutionize Diagnostics, Prognostics, and Treatment

AI technologies offer the potential to significantly enhance diagnostic accuracy, accelerate diagnostic timelines, and facilitate earlier disease detection across a wide spectrum of medical conditions, including cancer, cardiovascular diseases, and neurological disorders [8]. A key area of impact is personalized medicine, where AI can contribute by tailoring treatments to individual patient characteristics, derived from their unique data profiles [2]. For instance, AI models can predict how an individual patient might respond to specific therapies, such as chemotherapy or radiation, thereby guiding more effective and less toxic treatment selections [5]. Furthermore, AI can play a crucial role in reducing human error in data-intensive tasks like processing and analytics, achieved through automation and the consistent application of algorithmic processes [4].

Despite this transformative potential, the widespread integration of AI into routine clinical practice faces several challenges. These include addressing profound ethical implications related to data privacy, ensuring informed consent, and mitigating algorithmic bias [7]. Issues of data quality, accessibility, and standardization also pose significant hurdles, as does the complex task of integrating new AI technologies with pre-existing legacy healthcare systems and established clinical workflows [9]. The observation that clinicians require specific education and training to effectively use AI tools, and that the limitations of these tools must be thoroughly understood [2], signals an impending shift in medical education and continuous professional development. The introduction of AI into clinical settings is not merely about providing a new instrument; it necessitates a new paradigm of human-AI collaboration. Healthcare providers may find themselves needing to critically evaluate and integrate insights from AI programs that, in certain specialized areas, could possess a more extensive knowledge base than an individual clinician [9]. This evolving dynamic implies a change in the clinician's role from being the sole authority to becoming a skilled interpreter, critical appraiser, and responsible integrator of AI-generated information. Consequently, medical curricula will need to incorporate foundational knowledge in data science, AI principles, and the ethics of AI. Similarly, continuing medical education programs will need to address the emergence of new

AI tools, their appropriate applications, and their inherent limitations. This also carries significant implications for regulatory bodies and professional certification standards.

The current landscape of AI research in medicine is characterized by a dual focus: evaluating already existing applications for their clinical utility and safety, while simultaneously exploring the potential future roles of AI in virtually every field of clinical medicine [2]. This indicates a field that is concurrently striving to validate current tools for immediate, practical use and pushing the boundaries of innovation for long-term, transformative impact. This dynamic creates a productive tension and underscores the need for robust and standardized methodologies to assess both mature and emerging AI technologies. The development of comprehensive overviews and systematic reviews [2] is crucial in this context, as they help to map the current understanding, identify methodological best practices, and establish frameworks for comparing different AI applications, thereby providing structure to this rapidly evolving and impactful field.

3.3 Role of AI in Cancer Detection (General Oncology)

3.3.1 AI-Driven Advancements in Detecting Various Cancers

AI is fundamentally reshaping the landscape of oncological care. Its applications are leading to substantial improvements in cancer screening methodologies, the ability to predict disease progression with greater accuracy, the tailoring of therapeutic interventions to individual patient profiles, and an overall increase in workflow efficiency within clinical settings [3]. AI-powered tools have markedly advanced cancer diagnostics, frequently demonstrating sensitivity levels that match or even surpass those of human experts in the detection of various malignancies, including cervical, lung, skin, and breast cancer [5]. For example, the CheXNeXt system [10], a Convolutional Neural Network (CNN) designed for identifying lung pathologies in chest X-rays, exhibited significantly greater sensitivity in detecting masses and nodules compared to board-certified radiologists, while maintaining comparable specificity [5]. Furthermore, deep learning techniques have achieved considerable success in medical image-based cancer diagnosis across a range of tasks, such as image classification, reconstruction, lesion detection, segmentation, image registration, and image synthesis [6].

The consistent observation that AI systems can match or, in some specific diagnostic tasks, exceed the performance of human experts [5] suggests a future trajectory where AI may transition from a purely assistive role to that of a primary interpreter in certain well-defined clinical contexts. This is particularly relevant for high-volume screening procedures where efficiency and accuracy are paramount. Such a shift would have profound implications for the traditional roles and requisite training of medical specialists. For instance, AI has demonstrated high sensitivity for cervical intraepithelial neoplasia detection than manual reading [5], and IA algorithms in mammography can reduce radiologist workload and improve detection [11]. This potential evolution could lead to a restructuring of diagnostic workflows, where human experts like radiologists and pathologists might increasingly focus on more complex and ambiguous cases, quality assurance, and the critical integration of AI-derived findings into comprehensive patient management strategies, rather than dedicating extensive time to the primary interpretation of images for common screening tests. Consequently, medical training programs would need to adapt to prepare future specialists for this collaborative human-AI diagnostic environment.

3.3.2 Applications in Medical Imaging, Genomics, and Pathology

The impact of AI on the oncology is broadly evident across several key diagnostic domains:

- **Medical Imaging:** Computer-Aided Diagnosis (CAD) systems are a prominent application of AI in medical imaging. These systems are further categorized into CADe (computer-aided detection), which flags potential abnormalities, and CADx (computer-aided diagnosis), which assists in characterizing these findings and assessing malignancy likelihood [5]. CAD systems are employed to help physicians interpret a variety of medical images, including X-rays, Magnetic Resonance Imaging (MRI), Computed Tomography (CT) scans, and mammograms, by providing quantitative analyses of suspicious lesions [5]. AI algorithms within CAD systems can alleviate the burden of screening, for instance, by functioning as an automated second reader in mammography, thereby improving efficiency and potentially catching lesions missed by a single human reader [11]. Deep learning models, especially CNNs, have proven exceptionally adept at analyzing these medical images, aiding clinicians in the diagnosis of a wide array of cancers such as lung, rectal, pancreatic, gastric, prostate, brain, and breast cancer [6]. As an illustration of their capability, one CNN trained on D-SOC (Digital Screening for Ovarian Cancer) examination images achieved an overall accuracy of 82.9% for cancer detection [12].
- **Genomics and Molecular Oncology:** AI is revolutionizing molecular oncology by integrating and analyzing complex data from metabolomics, genomic sequencing (Next-Generation Sequencing—NGS), and medical imaging to comprehensively characterize molecular profiles of tumors. In some contexts, these AI-driven approaches are beginning to augment or replace traditional, more time-consuming gene sequencing laboratory procedures [5]. AI algorithms can sift through vast genomic datasets to identify specific cancer-causing mutations, predict tumor responses to targeted therapies, and uncover novel biomarkers [5].
- **Pathology:** In the realm of pathology, AI excels at analyzing histopathological images with remarkable precision and consistency. CNNs, for example, can be

trained to differentiate between benign and malignant lung cancer tissue with high accuracy, contributing to earlier and more reliable diagnoses [5]. Beyond image analysis, Recurrent Neural Networks (RNNs) are utilized in Natural Language Processing (NLP) applications to extract clinically relevant information embedded within unstructured text, such as cancer pathology reports, converting narrative data into structured, analyzable formats [5].

- **Multimodal Data Fusion:** A particularly powerful application of AI in oncology involves the integration of structured data (e.g., electronic health records, laboratory results), unstructured data (e.g., clinical notes, imaging reports), and multimodal fusion data, which combines inputs from diverse sources like radiology, histology, genomics, and proteomics [5]. This holistic approach, which synthesizes varied data streams, provides a richer and more comprehensive understanding of a patient's condition, thereby enhancing both diagnostic and prognostic accuracy [5]. The development of both predictive AI, which forecasts outcomes such as diagnosing cancer from scans, and generative AI, which can create novel outputs not explicitly present in the training data [11], points toward an increasingly multifaceted AI toolkit for oncology. While most current diagnostic AI applications are predictive, generative AI holds considerable potential. For instance, it could be used to synthesize realistic medical images for training purposes, particularly for rare cancers where large datasets are scarce, thereby addressing the "small dataset" problem highlighted as a challenge in AI development [6]. Furthermore, generative AI could simulate tumor evolution under various treatment scenarios, offering a sophisticated tool for personalizing medicine beyond simple predictive classifications.

The pronounced emphasis on AI's capacity to analyze "high-dimensional patient data" [11] and "multimodal fusion data" [5] underscores that one of AI's most significant strengths in oncology lies in its ability to achieve holistic data integration. This moves the field beyond the limitations of single-modality analysis toward a more comprehensive and nuanced view of the patient, an endeavor that often surpasses human cognitive limits due to the sheer volume and complexity of the data involved. AI's proficiency in synthesizing these disparate data sources is pivotal to unlocking its full power in personalized oncology. This, in turn, necessitates the development and implementation of robust data infrastructure, interoperability standards, and data governance frameworks to enable such sophisticated fusion and analysis. A direct consequence of this capability is that AI may uncover complex biomarker signatures and interrelationships within the data that are not apparent when analyzing individual data types in isolation, leading to novel diagnostic and therapeutic insights.

3.4 Role of AI in Cancer Detection (Oral Oncology)

Oral cancer, like other malignancies, benefits significantly from early and accurate detection. AI is progressively demonstrating its utility across various facets of oral cancer diagnosis, leveraging its analytical power to interpret complex data and provide actionable insights.

3.4.1 *Automated Image Analysis*

Automated image analysis stands as a cornerstone of AI's contribution to oral cancer detection. AI algorithms, particularly deep learning models such as Convolutional Neural Networks (CNNs), are adept at scrutinizing diverse medical images pertinent to oral cancer. These include clinical photographs, histopathological slides obtained from biopsies, autofluorescence images, and white light images. The overarching goals of this automated analysis are to enhance diagnostic accuracy, alleviate the workload of physicians, and critically, enable the detection of oral cancer at its earliest, most treatable stages [1].

- **Clinical Photographs:** AI models are trained to analyze clinical photographs, which can often be captured using standard digital cameras or even smartphones. These models perform tasks such as object detection (identifying and localizing suspicious lesions within the oral cavity), segmentation (precisely outlining the boundaries of these lesions), and classification (categorizing lesions as benign, premalignant, or malignant) [13]. Sophisticated CNN architectures like EfficientNetB0, various ResNet models (e.g., ResNet50, ResNet101), DenseNet architectures, and Swin Transformers have demonstrated commendable performance. For instance, studies have reported EfficientNetB0 achieving approximately 85% accuracy with an Area Under the Curve (AUC) between 0.91 and 0.92, while Swin Transformer models have shown performance metrics around 0.98 [13]. The advent of smartphone-based AI applications is particularly noteworthy, as it promises to make oral cancer screening more affordable and widely accessible, especially in resource-limited geographical areas or underserved populations [1].
- **Histopathological Images:** The analysis of histopathology slides remains the definitive gold standard for cancer diagnosis. However, this process is traditionally labor-intensive, time-consuming, and can be subject to inter-observer variability among pathologists [6]. AI offers the potential to automate and standardize this critical analysis. CNNs, including architectures such as InceptionResNet-v2, ResNet50, VGG16/19, various DenseNet models (e.g., DenseNet121, DenseNet169, and DenseNet201), and MobileNet, are extensively employed for feature extraction from histopathological images and subsequent classification of dysplasia (precancerous changes) and OSCC [14]. For example, ResNet50 achieved 96.6% accuracy in one study analyzing histopathological images [15],

while DenseNet variants have demonstrated training accuracies ranging from 85% to over 98% [16]. InceptionV3, recognized for its robust deep feature extraction capabilities, is often used independently or in combination with other models like MobileNet, achieving high classification rates (e.g., 94% in a hybrid model for photographic images, and 84% for CT image classification in oral cancer contexts) [17]. More recently, Vision Transformers (ViTs) are emerging as a powerful alternative or complement to CNNs. ViTs analyze images by dividing them into patches and using attention mechanisms to model long-range dependencies, thereby capturing global contextual relationships within tissue morphology. They are often fused with CNNs to further enhance performance in histopathological image analysis [14].

- **Autofluorescence and Other Imaging Modalities:** Beyond conventional photographs and histology, AI is also being applied to analyze images from other modalities. Autofluorescence imaging, which can highlight biochemical changes in tissues that may indicate malignancy, is one such area where AI interpretation can enhance detection capabilities [1]. Similarly, AI is being used to analyze Optical Coherence Tomography (OCT) images, which provide high-resolution, cross-sectional views of tissue, to improve the early detection of oral lesions [18].

Several CNN architectures have been prominently featured in oral cancer research due to their specific strengths:

- **ResNet (Residual Networks):** Models like ResNet50 and ResNet101 are frequently chosen for their capacity to effectively train very deep networks. They achieve this by incorporating "residual connections" or "skip connections," which help mitigate the vanishing gradient problem that can plague deep architectures. These models have demonstrated high accuracy in classifying OSCC from both histopathological images and clinical photographs [15]. For instance, ResNet50 achieved a 92.15% accuracy in one study for oral cancer detection and an even higher 96.6% accuracy in another histopathological analysis [19].
- **DenseNet (Densely Connected Convolutional Networks):** Architectures such as DenseNet121, DenseNet169, and DenseNet201 are characterized by their dense connectivity pattern, where each layer receives feature maps from all preceding layers. This design encourages feature reuse, improves gradient flow throughout the network, and often leads to strong performance with fewer parameters compared to other architectures of similar depth. DenseNet121, for example, achieved an impressive 99% accuracy for classifying oral lesions in one study [19] and 90.24% accuracy in a separate histopathology study.22 DenseNet169 achieved a high F1-score of 0.98 when analyzing photographic images of oral lesions [20].
- **InceptionV3:** This architecture, part of the Inception family of models, is known for its efficient use of computational resources and its multi-scale processing capabilities, achieved through "inception modules" that apply convolutions of different filter sizes in parallel. InceptionV3 is valued for robust feature extraction and has been applied to classify oral cancer from CT images (achieving 84%

accuracy) and has been combined with other models like MobileNet for analyzing photographic images, yielding accuracies around 94% [13].
- **MobileNet**: MobileNet is a lightweight CNN architecture specifically designed for mobile and embedded vision applications where computational resources are limited. It uses depth wise separable convolutions to reduce model size and computational cost, making it highly suitable for mHealth solutions and rapid, accessible screening tools for oral cancer [15]. It is often used in combination with more complex models or as a standalone for preliminary screening.
- **VGGNet (VGG16, VGG19):** These are relatively simpler but deeper architectures (16 and 19 layers, respectively) that have historically performed well and have served as a common backbone for transfer learning in many computer vision tasks. In oral cancer detection, VGG19 achieved 96.26% accuracy with data augmentation in one histopathology study 22 and 98% accuracy on photographic images in another [13].
- **Vision Transformers (ViT):** Representing a newer paradigm in image analysis, ViTs treat an image as a sequence of patches and apply transformer encoder mechanisms, originally developed for NLP, to capture global relationships between these patches using self-attention. They have shown considerable promise in medical imaging, including oral cancer histopathology, often being fused with CNNs to leverage the local feature extraction strengths of CNNs and the global context modeling of ViTs [14].

To provide a clearer overview of the performance of these diverse AI models in oral cancer image analysis, Table 3.1 consolidates reported metrics from various studies. This allows for a more direct comparison of different AI approaches, their target image modalities, tasks, and their reported efficacy, facilitating a critical appraisal of the current state-of-the-art and identifying areas for future research.

3.4.2 Computer-Aided Diagnosis (CAD)

Computer-Aided Diagnosis (CAD) systems leverage AI algorithms to serve as an adjunctive tool for clinicians, primarily in the interpretation of medical images. The core philosophy of CAD is to provide a "second opinion" or to highlight areas of potential concern that warrant further human expert review, rather than to replace the clinician entirely [5]. These systems aim to improve diagnostic accuracy, enhance consistency among readers, and increase the overall efficiency of the diagnostic workflow. CAD systems are generally differentiated into two main types:

- **CADe (Computer-Aided Detection):** These systems are designed to detect potential abnormalities or suspicious lesions within medical images [5]. In the context of oral cancer, a CADe system might automatically flag regions in a clinical photograph, an autofluorescence image, or a radiological scan that exhibit characteristics suggestive of a lesion, thereby drawing the clinician's attention to these specific areas for closer inspection.

Table 3.1 Comparative performance of selected AI models in oral cancer image analysis

AI model/architecture	Image modality	Task	Key performance metrics (accuracy, sensitivity, specificity, AUC, F1-score)	Dataset size/ nature (if available)
ResNet50 [15]	Histopathology	Classification (benign vs. malignant)	Accuracy: 96.6%, Pre: 97%, Rec: 96%	OSCC images, binary classification
ResNet101 [13]	Clinical photographs	Classification (referral categories)	Training Acc: 78.30% (for referral vs. non-referral)	N/A
DenseNet121 [19]	Clinical photographs (oral lesions)	Classification	Acc: 99%, Sens: 100%, F1: 99%	700 oral photographs (350 OSCC, 350 normal)
DenseNet121 [19]	Histopathology (OSCC)	Classification	Acc: 90.24%, F1: 90.45%	5192 images (Normal and OSCC)
DenseNet169 [13]	Clinical photographs (oral lesions)	Classification (multiclass)	F1-score: 0.98	980 oral photographic images (3 classes)
InceptionV3 (improved) [21]	CT images	Classification (oral cancer vs. cyst)	Acc: 84.05%, Sens: 82.36%, Spec: 84.51%	2810 CT images (1578 cancer, 1232 cyst)
InceptionV3 & MobileNet (hybrid) [17]	Clinical photographs	Classification	Acc: 94%	N/A
EfficientNetB0 [13]	Clinical photographs	Classification (suspicious vs. benign)	Mean Acc: 85%, Mean Spec: 84.5%, Mean Sens: 86.7%, AUC: 0.911–0.92	~716 images (236 suspicious, 480 benign)
VGG19 [13]	Clinical photographs	Classification (benign vs. precancerous)	Acc: 98%, Spec: 97%, Sens: 89%	200 photographic images
InceptionResNet-v2 & ViT (SVM fusion) [14]	Histopathology (dysplasia)	Classification	Superior balanced accuracy, sensitivity, precision, AUC (compared to individual models)	237 images (leukoplakia w/& w/o dysplasia, OSCC)

- **CADx (Computer-Aided Diagnosis):** These systems extend beyond mere detection. Once a potential lesion is identified (either by a human or a CADe system), CADx tools assist in characterizing the lesion, often by providing a quantitative assessment of the likelihood of malignancy or by classifying the lesion type [5].

In the specific domain of oral and head and neck cancer (HNC), CAD models are actively being developed and researched for early-stage cancer detection. These models are trained on various medical imaging data, including CT scans, MRI, and Positron Emission Tomography (PET) scans, with the objective of automatically identifying worrisome lesions or areas that are suggestive of cancer [22]. An emerging and promising area is the integration of Hyperspectral Imaging (HSI) with CAD techniques for enhanced HNC detection. HSI captures detailed spectral information beyond what is visible to the human eye or standard cameras, and AI algorithms such as Linear Discriminant Analysis (LDA), CNNs, and SVMs are being applied to analyze this rich HSI data [22]. A meta-analysis focusing on HSI for HNC reported varying performance among these algorithms, with LDA achieving an accuracy of 92%, CNNs 82%, and SVMs 76% [22]. The fundamental goal remains for CAD to be a complementary technology that augments the capabilities of physicians, rather than a system that operates with complete autonomy in making final diagnostic decisions [23].

3.4.3 Risk Stratification

AI models are increasingly being developed for risk stratification in oral cancer. The primary objective of these models is twofold: to identify individuals within a population who are at a heightened risk of developing oral cancer in the first place, and to predict the likelihood of malignant transformation in patients who present with Oral Potentially Malignant Disorders (OPMDs), as well as to forecast the risk of disease recurrence in patients who have previously been treated for oral cancer [1]. To achieve these predictive capabilities, AI-driven risk stratification models leverage a diverse array of data inputs [13]:

- **Clinical and Demographic Information:** This includes patient age, gender, lifestyle risk factors (such as tobacco and alcohol use), family history of cancer, and other relevant medical history data, often extracted from patient records.
- **Histopathological Descriptors:** Features derived from the microscopic examination of biopsy tissues, such as the grade of dysplasia, cellular atypia, and architectural changes, are critical inputs.
- **Standardized Images:** This encompasses various imaging modalities, including clinical photographs of oral lesions and high-resolution Whole Slide Images (WSIs) of histopathological samples.

- **Combined Data Types:** Often, the most robust risk stratification models integrate information from multiple sources, combining clinical, demographic, histopathological, and imaging data to create a comprehensive risk profile.

Various methodologies are employed in these models. Artificial Neural Networks (ANNs) and Natural Language Processing (NLP) techniques have been used to predict OSCC risk from clinical and demographic data, with some studies reporting accuracies around 78% [13]. Image-based risk stratification using CNNs, such as InceptionV3 applied to WSIs, has achieved high accuracy (e.g., 95.4%) in predicting the malignant transformation of OPMDs [13]. Pathomics-based models, which extract quantitative features from H&E-stained images, have also demonstrated strong predictive performance, with AUC values ranging from 0.8 to 0.9 [13]. Furthermore, machine learning techniques like random forest classifiers and sophisticated survival models (e.g., DeepSurv) are utilized to integrate multimodal data, assess cancer risk, and thereby support personalized care strategies [18].

The impact of accurate risk stratification is significant. By providing insights into which patients face a greater likelihood of malignancy development or disease recurrence, these AI tools can facilitate the delivery of personalized care. This may involve tailored screening intervals, prophylactic interventions for high-risk OPMDs, or more intensive surveillance protocols for post-treatment patients, ultimately aiming to improve patient prognosis and long-term outcomes [13].

3.4.4 Integration with Electronic Health Records (EHR)

The integration of AI with Electronic Health Records (EHR) holds a substantial promise for enhancing the detection, risk prediction, and overall management of oral cancer. AI algorithms can meticulously analyze the vast and diverse repositories of patient data stored within EHR systems. This data typically includes patient demographics, comprehensive medical histories, laboratory test results, unstructured clinical notes, medication records, and documented risk factors [9]. The benefits of such AI-EHR integration, while discussed in a general healthcare context, are directly applicable and highly relevant to oral oncology [24]:

- **Improved Diagnostic Accuracy and Complication Prediction:** AI can process longitudinal patient data from EHRs to identify subtle patterns or trends that may indicate an increased risk of oral cancer or predict potential complications related to the disease or its treatment.
- **Streamlined Patient Record Management and Administrative Efficiency:** AI tools, particularly those leveraging Natural Language Processing (NLP), can extract structured information from unstructured clinical notes within EHRs. Speech recognition can facilitate more efficient data entry, thereby reducing the administrative burden on clinicians and allowing them more time for direct patient care.

- **Enhanced Diagnostic Support:** AI systems integrated with EHRs can provide smart diagnostic suggestions to clinicians. These suggestions can be based on an analysis of listed symptoms, interpretations of medical images (if linked to the EHR), lab test results, and other patient data, helping to flag potential oral cases earlier.
- **Personalized Treatment Planning:** By identifying patterns in a patient's symptoms, genetic predispositions (if available in the EHR), and previous test results, AI can assist in tailoring treatment plans more precisely to the individual patient.

Specific to oral cancer, one study highlighted the use of 26 features extracted from EHRs to train machine learning algorithms for predicting the risk of malignant transformation in OPMDs [25]. Another study by Alhazmi (2021) developed an Artificial Neural Network (ANN) model that utilized data on risk factors, systemic medical conditions, and clinicopathological features, information typically found within or like EHR data to predict an individual's risk of developing oral cancer [25].

Despite these potential benefits, significant challenges persist. Healthcare data within EHRs is often fragmented, residing in disparate systems with varying formats. This lack of interoperability and consistency can create substantial issues regarding the completeness and accuracy of data required for training effective AI models [9]. Furthermore, the "dataset ceiling effect" [7], previously discussed, is particularly pertinent here. If AI models are trained on EHR data that contains undiagnosed or miscoded conditions, or inherent biases in documentation, the AI may learn and perpetuate these inaccuracies.

3.4.5 Prediction Models

AI-driven prediction models are being developed to forecast a wide range of aspects related to oral cancer. These models aim to predict the incidence of oral cancer in specific populations, the likely progression of OPMDs, the probability of malignant transformation of these precursor lesions, and the risk of postoperative recurrence in patients who have undergone treatment [1].

The methodologies employed for these prediction models are diverse, encompassing both traditional machine learning techniques and more complex deep learning approaches. Commonly used machine learning algorithms include Support Vector Machines (SVMs), Random Forest classifiers, and Multilayer Perceptrons (MLPs) [13]. Deep learning models, particularly various forms of neural networks, are also extensively used. The inputs for these models can be varied, often drawing from clinical data (patient history, risk factors), histopathological features extracted from biopsy samples, imaging data (such as features from clinical photographs or radiological scans), or, increasingly, a combination of these multimodal data sources to create more robust and accurate predictions [13]. For instance, one study demonstrated that an MLP model exhibited good sensitivity in predicting the postoperative recurrence of oral cancer, with the model performing best when provided with a comprehensive set of input variables rather than a more limited set of characteristic variables [26].

The impact of developing accurate and reliable prediction models for oral cancer is profound. Such models can lead to more personalized surveillance strategies, allowing clinicians to tailor the frequency and intensity of follow-up based on an individual's predicted risk. They can also inform decisions about the necessity and timing of interventions, particularly for OPMDs with a high predicted risk of transformation. Ultimately, effective prediction models contribute to improved patient outcomes by enabling proactive management and earlier detection of adverse events like recurrence [13]. Indeed, AI models have demonstrated the potential to outperform existing clinical approaches in predicting the occurrence and course of oral cancer [27].

3.4.6 Mobile Health (mHealth) Solutions

Mobile Health (mHealth) solutions, leveraging the ubiquity of smartphones and the power of AI, are emerging as a significant avenue for making oral cancer screening, awareness campaigns, and early detection efforts more accessible and affordable. This is particularly crucial in resource-constrained settings or geographically remote areas where access to specialized dental and medical care is limited [1]. The functionality of these mHealth applications is varied and innovative:

- **Guided Self-Examination and Image Capture:** Many apps are designed to guide users through systematic oral self-examinations. They can then utilize the smartphone's camera to capture images of the oral cavity. Integrated AI algorithms subsequently analyze these images to identify any suspicious lesions or abnormalities that may warrant further professional attention [28].
- **Educational Content and Gamification:** To enhance user engagement and knowledge, some mHealth apps incorporate educational videos, interactive content, and "serious games" (games designed for a primary purpose other than pure entertainment). These elements aim to improve awareness about oral cancer, its risk factors, signs and symptoms, and the importance of prevention and early detection [29].
- **Teleconsultation Capabilities:** Certain mHealth platforms facilitate teleconsultation by enabling users or local healthcare workers to securely transmit clinical data and images of oral lesions to dentists or specialists for remote review and consultation. This can bridge geographical barriers and expedite access to expert opinions [27].

The effectiveness and feasibility of such mHealth AI solutions are supported by emerging research. For example, a study involving the TEGO® (Tele-platform of Geriatric and Dental Specialties App) in Chile demonstrated that its use significantly increased oral cancer awareness and the practice of oral self-examinations among older adults [30]. Similarly, the MeMoSA (Mobile Mouth Screening App) study in Malaysia showcased the feasibility of using an mHealth application for oral cancer screening in rural communities, conducted by trained healthcare volunteers, achieving a high uptake rate of 93% [27]. This study also identified key facilitators, such as the ease of use of the app, cost savings for patients (by avoiding travel to clinics), and the trust established with community leaders. However, it also highlighted barriers, including limitations in internet infrastructure in remote areas and community perceptions or fear surrounding cancer screening [27].

The significance of AI-powered mHealth solutions lies in their potential to democratize access to early screening for oral cancer. By bringing diagnostic support directly to individuals or primary healthcare workers via readily available technology, these tools can help shift the detection of oral cancer to earlier, more treatable stages. This is particularly impactful for underserved populations who face the greatest barriers to accessing traditional healthcare services, potentially leading to a reduction in oral cancer disparities and an improvement in overall survival rates [1].

The convergence of automated image analysis (especially CNNs adept at interpreting clinical photographs), the principles of CAD systems, and the widespread accessibility of mHealth platforms creates a powerful synergy. This combination has the potential to revolutionize oral cancer screening by decentralizing it, making it low-cost, and scalable. It's not merely about the advancement of individual technologies but their combined capacity to shift the paradigm of screening from specialized, often reactive, clinical settings to proactive community-based or even home-based initiatives. Such a transformation could dramatically improve early detection rates on a population scale, particularly in low- and middle-income countries where the burden of oral cancer is often highest and resources are most scarce.

Furthermore, the ability of AI to integrate diverse data types ranging from clinical and demographic information often found in EHRs, to imaging data from various modalities, and detailed histopathological findings for comprehensive risk stratification and the development of sophisticated prediction models points toward a future of highly personalized oral cancer prevention and management. This moves beyond the reactive detection of existing cancer to a proactive approach focused on identifying individuals at high risk and managing that risk effectively before cancer develops or recurs. This could be manifested in dynamic, individualized risk scores that trigger personalized screening schedules, tailored prophylactic advice, or more intensive and targeted follow-up protocols for patients' post-treatment, thereby significantly improving long-term outcomes and potentially even reducing the overall incidence of oral cancer.

Underlying these specific applications is a recurring theme: AI systems frequently demonstrate performance that either matches or surpasses traditional diagnostic and prognostic approaches or significantly augments human capabilities [1]. This suggests a fundamental technological shift, where AI is not merely offering incremental improvements but is acting as a disruptive technology that challenges and has the potential to redefine established paradigms in oral oncology. This consistent trend of outperformance or augmentation across diverse AI applications from image analysis and CAD to risk stratification and predictive modeling signals is a compelling need for the dental and medical professions to actively engage with, rigorously validate, and thoughtfully integrate these AI tools into clinical practice. Resistance to adoption could inadvertently mean missing significant opportunities for improving patient care and outcomes. Concurrently, ethical guidelines and regulatory frameworks must evolve at a commensurate pace to accommodate this disruptive potential responsibly, ensuring that patient safety, data privacy, and equity remain paramount.

3.5 Various Stages of Detection and Diagnosis of Oral Cancer Using AI

Artificial intelligence is being applied across the entire spectrum of oral cancer detection and diagnosis, from initial population screening to detailed pathological assessment and treatment planning. Its role evolves depending on the specific clinical question and the data available at each stage.

3.5.1 Screening and Triage

AI plays a crucial role in the initial stages of oral cancer detection, particularly in screening programs and patient triage. The aim is to develop automated systems that can identify suspicious lesions at an early stage, often utilizing readily accessible data modalities like clinical photographs [1]. This is especially valuable for screening high-risk populations or for use in settings where access to specialist oral healthcare professionals is limited [25]. Photography-based AI models are considered ideal for such scenarios due to their potential for low-cost, non-invasive screening [13]. For instance, AI systems can analyze images captured by simple smartphone probes, making screening feasible even in remote or inaccessible regions [25].

Beyond initial detection, AI assists in the critical task of patient triage. By classifying identified lesions based on their likelihood of malignancy, AI can help facilitate appropriate and timely referral of patients from primary care settings to specialists [13]. This optimizes the use of specialist resources and ensures that individuals with high-risk lesions receive expert consultation without undue delay. It has been observed that general dentists may sometimes lack a consistent and analytical decision-making strategy when differentiating between malignant, premalignant, and benign oral epithelial lesions based solely on clinical cues; AI can serve as a valuable adjunctive tool to improve this triage accuracy [25]. AI models for triage can range from binary classification systems (e.g., "referral warranted" vs. "no referral needed") to more complex multiclass discriminative tasks that provide more nuanced risk assessments [13].

3.5.2 *Histopathology Image Analysis*

The histopathological examination of a tissue biopsy remains the definitive gold standard for the diagnosis of oral cancer. However, this process is traditionally labor-intensive, requires significant expertise, can be time-consuming, and is susceptible to inter-observer variability among pathologists [6]. AI is being increasingly applied to automate, standardize, and enhance this critical diagnostic step. Key applications of AI in histopathology image analysis for oral cancer include:

- **Dysplasia Detection and Grading:** AI models, predominantly CNNs and, more recently, Vision Transformers (ViTs), are trained to classify histopathological images to detect the presence of dysplasia (precancerous changes) and to grade its severity. Dysplasia grading is a critical indicator of the potential for progression to invasive oral cancer [1].
- **Malignancy Identification:** A core task is the differentiation of benign lesions from malignant ones (OSCC) within biopsy samples [15]. AI algorithms can identify subtle morphological and architectural variations within the tissue that are indicative of cellular abnormalities and malignancy [14].
- **Automated Feature Extraction:** Deep learning models excel at automatically extracting hierarchical and often complex features directly from the image data. These learned features are then used for classification, eliminating the need for manual feature engineering which can be subjective and incomplete [6].
- **Segmentation:** AI is used for segmentation tasks, such as accurately identifying and delineating individual nuclei or entire tumor regions within Whole Slide Images (WSIs). This quantitative information can be valuable for assessing tumor characteristics and heterogeneity [6].

Numerous studies have reported high performance for AI models in diagnosing, classifying, and predicting oral cancer from histopathological images, with accuracies often ranging from 89% to 100% [22]. These systems have the potential to outperform existing clinical approaches in certain tasks, reduce the workload of pathologists, and improve diagnostic consistency [1]. For example, a fusion model combining features extracted by InceptionResNet-v2 and a ViT, subsequently classified by SVMs, demonstrated superior performance in classifying oral dysplasia compared to individual models [14].

3.5.3 *Prognosis and Risk Analysis*

Beyond the initial diagnosis, AI models are being developed to analyze a confluence of clinical, histopathological, and imaging data to predict patient prognosis. This includes forecasting survival rates, estimating the likelihood of disease recurrence after treatment, and determining the probability of malignant transformation of OPMDs [1]. Machine learning techniques such as random forest classifiers and specialized survival models like DeepSurv are employed to integrate these multimodal data sources, thereby providing individualized risk assessments that can guide clinical management [18]. Furthermore, AI can assist in identifying novel prognostic biomarkers from complex datasets, such as patterns in metabolomic profiles (e.g., uracil levels) that correlate with patient outcomes [31]. The ability to accurately predict prognosis and analyze risk is crucial for tailoring follow-up schedules, making informed decisions regarding the necessity of adjuvant therapies, and managing patient expectations effectively.

3.5.4 Treatment Planning and Response Monitoring

AI is also making inroads into the domains of treatment planning and monitoring treatment response in oral cancer. For personalized treatment strategies, AI algorithms assist in formulating individualized treatment plans by processing and integrating multimodal patient information. This includes data on the clinical stage of cancer, tumor dimensions, specific site, histopathological grade, and molecular profiles (e.g., genomic or proteomic data) [1]. AI can predict how an individual patient might respond to different therapeutic modalities, such as chemotherapy or radiation therapy, thereby helping to select the most effective treatment while minimizing potential toxicity [5]. AI-driven Clinical Decision Support Systems (AI-CDSS) can further optimize treatment plans by considering unique patient parameters, tumor characteristics, and identified risk factors [1].

In terms of tracking efficacy (response monitoring), AI offers innovative solutions. It can be utilized for real-time monitoring of patient vitals and assessing treatment response through various data streams [5]. For example, AI-powered biosensors are being conceptualized that could enable continuous, non-invasive monitoring of specific biomarkers (like uracil levels in saliva or plasma) to provide real-time insights into OSCC progression and the effectiveness of ongoing treatment [31]. Moreover, AI can analyze serial imaging data (e.g., CT scans, Immunohistochemistry (IHC) stained slides) obtained over the course of treatment to quantitatively assess changes in tumor size, morphology, or biomarker expression, thereby providing objective measures of treatment response [28].

3.5.5 Clinical Decision Support

Artificial Intelligence-based Clinical Decision Support Systems (AI-CDSS) represent a sophisticated application of AI, designed to integrate and analyze vast quantities of multimodal data to furnish clinicians with actionable insights and evidence-based recommendations for oral cancer management [1]. These systems typically process data from clinical images, patient histories (often from EHRs), molecular profiles, and pathology reports. The functionalities of AI-CDSS in oral cancer are diverse and impactful [1]:

- They facilitate early detection by flagging suspicious cases, enable more precise staging of the disease, and support the development of personalized treatment plans.
- AI-CDSS can interpret complex clinical results, identify critical disease patterns and correlations within the data, and help construct comprehensive patient profiles that offer a holistic view of the individual's condition.
- These systems can assist in grading and classifying oral cancer lesions, which is crucial information for effective treatment planning and accurate prognosis prediction.
- Drawing from broader AI-EHR capabilities, AI-CDSS could also offer suggestions for medication alternatives (considering allergies or drug interactions), calculate appropriate medication dosages, or recommend additional diagnostic tests based on the patient's overall health status and risk factors [24].

The implementation of AI-CDSS has the potential to significantly reduce diagnostic delays, improve the outcomes of interventions, optimize treatment plans for individual efficacy, and enhance the overall accuracy of diagnosis in oral cancer [31]. Preliminary studies evaluating deep learning algorithms within CDSS frameworks for oral cancer have reported promisingly high accuracy rates [32].

The role of AI demonstrably evolves across this diagnostic continuum. It begins with broad, accessible applications in screening and triage, often leveraging easily obtainable data like clinical photographs processed by mHealth solutions. It then transitions to highly specialized and detailed analyses, such as the automated interpretation of histopathological slides, which requires sophisticated image processing and pattern recognition. Finally, it culminates in complex data integration for personalized treatment planning and ongoing clinical decision support. This progression indicates that AI is not a monolithic solution but rather a versatile and adaptable toolkit. Its various components can be tailored to address the different stages and inherent complexities of the oral cancer care pathway, from initial suspicion to long-term management. The successful integration of AI into comprehensive oral cancer care will therefore likely require a suite of distinct AI tools, each optimized for specific tasks, data types, and clinical questions, rather than a single, all-encompassing approach. This also underscores a future need for interoperability between these tools to ensure seamless data flow and integrated decision-making.

Furthermore, an emerging trend, particularly evident in histopathology image analysis and treatment response monitoring, is the combination of AI with novel imaging or sensing technologies. Examples include the use of AI with Hyperspectral Imaging (HSI) in Head and Neck Cancer (a field closely related to oral cancer) [22] and the conceptualization of AI-powered biosensors for monitoring biomarkers like uracil [31]. This suggests a future where AI not only enhances the analysis of existing data types but also becomes instrumental in unlocking the clinical utility of new, information-rich diagnostic modalities. These next-generation technologies often generate data of such complexity and volume that it might be overwhelming or impractical for human interpretation alone. AI could thus be the key to translating these advanced diagnostic capabilities into tangible clinical benefits, leading to even earlier and more precise detection and monitoring by making sense of data streams that are currently underutilized or too intricate for manual analysis.

It is also crucial to recognize that the effectiveness of an overarching AI-clinical decision support system is directly contingent upon the quality, accuracy, and robustness of the AI applications that feed into it from the preceding stages of screening, image analysis, and prognostic modeling. If the AI-driven tools used for initial screening, histopathological interpretation, or risk prediction are flawed, contain biases, or lack generalizability, the decision support offered by the integrated CDSS will inevitably be compromised. The principle of "garbage in, garbage out" is highly relevant here. Therefore, if the AI components that provide input to the CDSS are inaccurate or biased, the recommendations generated by the CDSS will reflect these underlying flaws. This highlights the paramount importance of rigorous validation, meticulous bias mitigation strategies, and continuous performance monitoring for all AI tools deployed across the entire diagnostic pipeline, as errors or shortcomings in one component can compound and negatively impact subsequent decisions. It also emphasizes the need for transparency and explainability in how AI-CDSS systems arrive at their recommendations, allowing clinicians to understand the basis of the advice and critically evaluate its applicability to the individual patient.

3.6 Challenges, Limitations, and Future Outlook

Despite the significant promise of AI in revolutionizing oral cancer detection, its widespread and effective clinical integration is contingent upon addressing a range of multifaceted challenges and limitations. Understanding these hurdles is crucial for guiding future research and development efforts.

3.6.1 Current Hurdles

- **Data Quality, Quantity, and Accessibility:** A primary and recurrent limitation in the development of robust AI models for oral pathology is the scarcity of large, high-quality, well-annotated, and diverse datasets [1]. Training effective deep learning models typically requires substantial amounts of data to learn complex patterns and generalize well. Variability in tissue fixation, slide preparation, staining procedures, and image acquisition protocols across different institutions can introduce inconsistencies that negatively impact AI model performance [33]. Furthermore, the limited availability of publicly accessible, standardized datasets hinders collaborative research, benchmarking of new algorithms, and independent validation of published models [6]. This is particularly acute for rare subtypes of oral cancer or less common OPMDs.

- **Model Generalizability and Robustness:** AI models, especially those trained on data from a single institution or a limited demographic, often struggle to generalize their performance accurately when applied to new, unseen data from different patient cohorts, clinical settings, or imaging devices [6]. This lack of generalizability means a model that performs well in a research setting may falter in real-world clinical practice. Overfitting, where a model learns the training data too well, including its noise and specific biases, but fails to perform adequately on external data, is a common issue that needs careful mitigation [6].
- **Algorithmic Bias:** A significant concern is the potential for algorithmic bias. If the datasets used to train AI models are not representative of the diverse populations in which these tools will be deployed (e.g., underrepresentation of certain skin tones in clinical photographs, or specific age groups or ethnicities), the models may perform less accurately or unfairly for these underrepresented groups [1]. This could inadvertently exacerbate existing health disparities rather than alleviating them [34].
- **Interpretability and Explainability (The "Black Box" Problem):** Many advanced AI models, particularly deep learning networks, operate as "black boxes." Their internal decision-making processes can be opaque and difficult for humans to understand [6]. This lack of transparency is a major barrier to clinical trust and adoption, as clinicians need to understand why an AI system arrives at a particular diagnosis or recommendation to confidently integrate it into patient care and to identify potential errors [18].
- **Integration into Clinical Workflows:** Successfully embedding AI tools into existing, often complex, healthcare systems and established clinical workflows present considerable technical and logistical challenges [1]. This requires not only technological compatibility but also adaptation by healthcare professionals, who need adequate training and support to use these new technologies effectively and appropriately [1].

Many of these challenges are deeply interconnected. For instance, the lack of high-quality, diverse datasets [33] not only directly impedes model performance in terms of accuracy and generalizability [6] but can also be a primary source of algorithmic bias if the available data does not reflect the target population [9]. This bias, in turn, raises significant ethical concerns regarding fairness and equity in healthcare delivery [33]. Therefore, addressing one challenge, such as improving data quality, often requires a concomitant consideration of its impact on other related issues, like bias mitigation and model robustness. Solutions must be holistic; focusing solely on algorithmic improvements without fundamentally addressing underlying data issues will likely yield limited and potentially flawed success.

3.6.2 *Ethical, Legal, and Regulatory Landscape*

The deployment of AI in oral cancer detection also navigates a complex ethical, legal, and regulatory terrain [9]:

- **Data Privacy and Security:** The use of sensitive patient data for training and validating AI models necessitates strict adherence to data privacy regulations, such as the Health Insurance Portability and Accountability Act (HIPAA) in the United States, to protect patient confidentiality.
- **Accountability and Liability:** Establishing clear lines of accountability and liability in cases where AI-generated diagnoses or recommendations lead to errors or adverse patient outcomes is a critical and unresolved issue.
- **Informed Consent:** Ethical considerations surrounding patient consent for the use of their data in AI development and application are paramount, ensuring patients are adequately informed about how their information will be utilized.
- **Regulatory Approval:** AI tools intended for clinical use, especially diagnostic aids, must undergo rigorous validation and obtain approval from regulatory bodies (e.g., FDA in the US, EMA in Europe). This process can be lengthy, complex and requires clear evidence of safety and efficacy [33]. There is a growing recognition of the need for standardized reporting guidelines for AI studies in medicine, such as TRIPOD-AI and CONSORT-AI [8], to ensure transparency and facilitate robust evaluation.

The rapid pace of AI development [6] often outstrips the evolution of corresponding ethical guidelines, regulatory frameworks [9], and comprehensive clinical validation processes, including essential longitudinal studies [1]. This creates a potential "pace problem" a gap where powerful AI tools might become technologically available before their safe, ethical, and effective use in diverse real-world clinical settings is fully established and understood. This situation necessitates proactive and anticipatory engagement from ethicists, policymakers, healthcare organizations, and clinical bodies. The goal should be to develop "agile governance" frameworks that can adapt to ongoing technological advancements while steadfastly ensuring patient safety, upholding ethical principles, and promoting equitable access to beneficial AI innovations.

3.6.3 *Financial Constraints*

The implementation and maintenance of AI systems in oral pathology and broader oncological settings can be financially demanding [33]. Costs are associated with setting up the necessary infrastructure (hardware, software, and data storage), acquiring or developing AI models, integrating them into existing systems, ongoing maintenance and updates, and the training of personnel to use these advanced systems effectively [33]. The high cost of some AI-powered healthcare tools can also limit accessibility, particularly in low-resource settings or for underinsured populations, potentially widening health disparities [34].

3.6.4 Emerging Trends and Future Directions

Despite the challenges, the field is actively pursuing several promising future directions:

- **Explainable AI (XAI):** There is strong research emphasis on developing XAI methods. Techniques such as LIME (Local Interpretable Model-agnostic Explanations), SHAP (SHapley Additive exPlanations), and Class Activation Mapping (CAM) aim to make the decision-making processes of AI models more transparent and interpretable [6]. This is crucial for fostering clinical trust, facilitating error analysis, and ensuring responsible AI deployment.
- **Multimodal Data Integration:** Future AI models will increasingly leverage the power of multimodal data, integrating diverse sources such as imaging (clinical photos, CT, MRI, HSI, OCT), genomics, proteomics, metabolomics, clinical records from EHRs, and pathology reports to build more comprehensive, robust, and accurate diagnostic and prognostic systems [5].
- **Federated Learning:** This approach allows AI models to be trained across multiple institutions or datasets without requiring the raw patient data to leave its original location. Instead, model updates are shared, addressing privacy concerns while enabling access to larger and more diverse datasets for training more generalizable models.
- **Development of Public Standard Databases:** The creation and curation of large, high-quality, publicly available, and standardized databases for oral cancer (and other cancers) are recognized as critical for benchmarking new algorithms, fostering reproducible research, and accelerating progress in the field [6].
- **Longitudinal Studies:** There is a pressing need for more longitudinal studies to validate the performance and clinical impact of AI models over extended periods in real-world clinical settings. This will provide crucial evidence on their long-term reliability and utility [1].
- **Advanced Neural Networks and Hybrid Models:** Research continues into refining existing neural network architectures and exploring novel ones, including further development of Vision Transformers (ViT), ensemble learning techniques (which combine multiple models to improve performance), and hybrid models that integrate different AI approaches (e.g., CNN-ViT fusions, AI with traditional ML classifiers) [6].
- **Few-Shot Learning:** Developing AI models that can be effectively learnt from smaller datasets (few-shot or zero-shot learning) is an important research direction, particularly relevant for rare cancer types or situations where extensive annotated data is inherently difficult to obtain [6].

While AI technologies aim to automate processes and augment human capabilities, the "human factor" remains a critical component for successful development and implementation. This includes the domain expertise required by pathologists and clinicians to accurately annotate data for training [6], the trust and acceptance needed from clinicians who will ultimately use these AI tools in their practice (which XAI aims to foster) [1], and the patients whose data fuels these systems and who are the ultimate beneficiaries of improved care. Overlooking this human element in the design, development, validation, and implementation of AI can lead to poor adoption rates, user dissatisfaction, or even unintended negative consequences. Therefore, successful AI integration is not merely a technical challenge but a socio-technical one. It demands user-centered design principles, continuous education and training for healthcare professionals, and a deeply collaborative approach involving AI developers, clinicians, ethicists, patients, and regulatory bodies to ensure that AI tools are not only accurate and efficient but also usable, trusted, aligned with clinical needs, and ethically deployed.

3.6.5 Recommendations for Advancing Research and Clinical Implementation

To harness the full potential of AI in oral cancer detection, a concerted effort is needed:

- Foster multi-institutional and international collaborations to facilitate data sharing (where ethically and legally permissible, perhaps via federated learning) and the creation of large, diverse datasets essential for training robust and generalizable AI models [33].
- Develop and adhere to standardized protocols for data collection, image acquisition, annotation, and the evaluation and reporting of AI model performance to ensure consistency and comparability across studies [1].
- Prioritize and invest in research focused on XAI techniques, methods for mitigating algorithmic bias, and strategies for enhancing the robustness and generalization of AI models across varied clinical contexts.
- Establish clear, adaptable, and internationally harmonized ethical guidelines and regulatory frameworks specifically tailored for the development, validation, and deployment of AI in healthcare, particularly for diagnostic applications.
- Promote comprehensive education and training programs for current and future healthcare professionals to improve AI literacy, enabling them to understand, critically appraise, and effectively utilize AI tools in their clinical practice.

Table 3.2 provides a structured summary of the key challenges facing the field and the corresponding future directions being pursued to overcome them.

Artificial intelligence is unequivocally demonstrating significant potential to transform the landscape of early detection and diagnosis of oral cancer. Through a

Table 3.2 Summary of key challenges and future directions for AI in oral cancer detection

Challenge/limitation category	Specific issue	Potential solutions/future research focus
Data-related [1, 6]	Small dataset size, lack of high-quality annotated data	Federated learning, multi-institutional data collaboratives, public standard databases, synthetic data generation (generative AI)
	Data heterogeneity and variability (acquisition, processing)	Standardized protocols for data collection & annotation, data harmonization techniques
	Limited accessibility to diverse datasets	Public dataset initiatives, data sharing agreements (with privacy safeguards)
Model-related [1, 6]	Lack of generalizability, overfitting	Training on diverse datasets, domain adaptation techniques, robust validation on external data, few-shot learning
	"Black box" nature, lack of interpretability	Explainable AI (XAI) methods (LIME, SHAP, CAM), inherently interpretable models
	Algorithmic bias leading to health disparities	Bias detection and mitigation techniques, training on representative and diverse data, fairness-aware AI design
Ethical/Regulatory [9]	Patient data privacy and security	Robust data governance, anonymization/de-identification techniques, federated learning, compliance with HIPAA/GDPR
	Accountability and liability for AI errors	Clear legal frameworks, defining roles and responsibilities in human–AI collaboration
	Need for regulatory approval and standards	Rigorous validation studies, standardized reporting guidelines (e.g., CONSORT-AI, TRIPOD-AI), agile regulatory pathways
Implementation/financial [1, 33]	Integration into clinical workflows	User-centered design, interoperability standards, pilot programs, clinician training
	Cost of development, deployment, and maintenance	Cost-benefit analyses, development of value-based AI solutions, open-source initiatives
	Need for healthcare professional training	AI literacy programs in medical education, continuous professional development on AI tools

diverse array of applications—including sophisticated automated image analysis of clinical photographs and histopathological slides, the development of Computer-Aided Diagnosis (CAD) systems to assist clinicians, advanced risk stratification models leveraging multimodal data, seamless integration with Electronic Health Records (EHR) for comprehensive patient data analysis, robust predictive modeling for forecasting disease incidence and recurrence, and innovative Mobile Health (mHealth) solutions for accessible screening AI is paving the way for substantial improvements. These advancements collectively promise enhanced diagnostic accuracy, increased operational efficiency in clinical workflows, greater accessibility to screening, particularly in underserved regions, and the facilitation of more personalized approaches to patient care in oral oncology.

The promising results reported in numerous studies underscore the tangible capabilities of AI in identifying oral cancer and its precursors with high levels of sensitivity and specificity, often comparable or even superior to traditional methods [1]. While significant challenges pertaining to data quality and accessibility, model robustness and generalizability, ethical considerations, and seamless clinical integration persist, the field is actively addressing these hurdles. Ongoing research and development, particularly in areas such as Explainable AI (XAI) to demystify "black box" models, advanced techniques for multimodal data fusion to create more holistic patient profiles, and concerted efforts toward the establishment of standardized, large-scale, and publicly available datasets are critical in paving the path toward broader and more confident clinical adoption. The ultimate objective is to translate the analytical power of AI into measurable improvements in patient outcomes, thereby contributing to a reduction in the global burden of oral cancer through earlier, more precise, and more equitable detection strategies.

The journey of AI in oral cancer detection is characterized by continuous innovation, which must be parallel by rigorous validation and a steadfast commitment to ethical principles. Realizing the full clinical potential of these powerful technologies will necessitate a sustained, multidisciplinary collaborative effort, bringing together AI researchers, data scientists, clinicians, pathologists, ethicists, regulatory bodies, and patient advocates. Such collaboration is essential to ensure that AI tools are developed and deployed responsibly, effectively, and equitably, ultimately serving the best interests of patients at risk of or affected by oral cancer. The overarching narrative is one of cautious optimism; while the potential of AI is immense and increasingly supported by empirical evidence, its successful and widespread clinical integration is contingent upon diligently and systematically overcoming the substantial, multifaceted challenges that lie ahead. The progress made in applying AI to oral cancer detection could also serve as a valuable model and provide impetus for the adoption of similar AI-driven strategies in the detection of other, perhaps less common or harder-to-diagnose, cancers, particularly those that could benefit from early visual recognition or complex data-pattern analysis. The lessons learned regarding dataset requirements, the importance of XAI, and effective integration strategies in oral cancer AI can contribute to a broader knowledge base and an expanding toolkit for AI in oncology, potentially accelerating progress across various cancer types.

References

1. Vinay, V., Jodalli, P., Chavan, M. S., Buddhikot, C. S., Luke, A. M., Ingafou, M. S. H., et al. (2025). Artificial intelligence in oral cancer: A comprehensive scoping review of diagnostic and prognostic applications. *Diagnostics, 15*(3), 280.
2. Morone, G., De Angelis, L., Cinnera, A. M., Carbonetti, R., Bisirri, A., Ciancarelli, I., et al. (2025). Artificial intelligence in clinical medicine: A state-of-the-art overview of systematic reviews with methodological recommendations for improved reporting. *Frontiers in Digital Health, 7*, 1550731.

3. Aftab, M., Mehmood, F., Zhang, C., Nadeem, A., Dong, Z., Jiang, Y., & Liu, K. (2025). AI in oncology: Transforming cancer detection through machine learning and deep learning applications. *arXiv preprint arXiv:2501.15489*
4. *What is Artificial Intelligence (AI)?* Retrieved May 2025, from https://cloud.google.com/learn/what-is-artificial-intelligence
5. Huhulea, E. N., Huang, L., Eng, S., Sumawi, B., Huang, A., Aifuwa, E., et al. (2025). Artificial intelligence advancements in oncology: A review of current trends and future directions. *Biomedicine, 13*(4), 951.
6. Jiang, X., Hu, Z., Wang, S., & Zhang, Y. (2023). Deep learning for medical image-based cancer diagnosis. *Cancer, 15*(14), 3608.
7. *AI on AI: Artificial intelligence in diagnostic medicine: Opportunities and challenges.* Retrieved May 2025, from https://armstronginstitute.blogs.hopkinsmedicine.org/2025/03/02/artificial-intelligence-in-diagnostic-medicine-opportunities-and-challenges/
8. Akhtar, Z. B. (2025). Artificial intelligence within medical diagnostics: A multi-disease perspective. *Artificial Intelligence in Health, 2*(3), 5173.
9. Alhejaily, A. M. G. (2025). Artificial intelligence in healthcare. *Biomedical Reports, 22*(1), 1–8.
10. *CheXNeXt: Deep learning for chest radiograph diagnosis.* Retrieved May 2025, from https://stanfordmlgroup.github.io/projects/chexnext/
11. Kolla, L., & Parikh, R. B. (2024). Uses and limitations of artificial intelligence for oncology. *Cancer, 130*(12), 2101–2107.
12. Ijaz, M. F., & Woźniak, M. (2024). Recent advances in deep learning and medical imaging for cancer treatment. *Cancer, 16*(4), 700.
13. Araújo, A. L. D., Pedroso, C. M., Vargas, P. A., Lopes, M. A., & Santos-Silva, A. R. (2025). Advancing oral cancer diagnosis and risk assessment with artificial intelligence: A review. *Exploration of Digital Health Technologies, 3*, 101147.
14. Pham, T. D. (2025). Integrating support vector machines and deep learning features for oral cancer histopathology analysis. *Biology Methods & Protocols, 10*(1), bpaf034.
15. Panigrahi, S., Nanda, B. S., Bhuyan, R., Kumar, K., Ghosh, S., & Swarnkar, T. (2023). Classifying histopathological images of oral squamous cell carcinoma using deep transfer learning. *Heliyon, 9*(3), e13444.
16. Redie, D. K., Bilgaiyan, S., & Sagnika, S. (2023). Oral cancer detection using transfer learning-based framework from histopathology images. *Journal of Electronic Imaging, 32*(5), 053004.
17. Sathishkumar, R., Harsavarthini, D., Agnes, C., & Jancy, R. (2025). Deep learning-driven oral cancer prediction using mobilenet and inception V3. *African Journal of Biomedical Research, 27*(4S), 15017–15025.
18. *AI and deep learning transform diagnosis of oral potentially malignant disorders.* Retrieved May 2025, from http://www.news-medical.net/news/20250226/AI-and-deep-learning-transform-diagnosis-of-oral-potentially-malignant-disorders.aspx
19. Süren, B., & Akar, M. (2025). Examination of ResNet and DenseNet architectures in early diagnosis of oral cancer: An evaluation. *Gazi University Journal of Science, 38*(2), 1006–1019.
20. Islam, S., Mahmud, M. Z., Alve, S. R., & Chowdhury, M. M. U. (2024). Deep learning approach for enhancing oral squamous cell carcinoma with LIME explainable AI technique. *arXiv preprint arXiv:2411.14184*
21. Xiang, S., He, Y., Huang, C., Guo, Z., Lin, S., & Zhu, J. (2023). A new intelligent model based on improved inception-V3 for oral cancer and cyst classification. *Journal of Mechanics in Medicine and Biology, 23*(09), 2340098.
22. Wu, I. C., Chen, Y. C., Karmakar, R., Mukundan, A., Gabriel, G., Wang, C. C., & Wang, H. C. (2024). Advancements in hyperspectral imaging and computer-aided diagnostic methods for the enhanced detection and diagnosis of head and neck cancer. *Biomedicine, 12*(10), 2315.
23. Doi, K. (2007). Computer-aided diagnosis in medical imaging: Historical review, current status and future potential. *Computerized Medical Imaging and Graphics, 31*(4–5), 198–211.
24. *Artificial Intelligence for EHR: Use cases, costs, challenges.* Sciencesoft. Retrieved May 2025, from https://www.scnsoft.com/healthcare/ehr/artificial-intelligence

25. Hegde, S., Ajila, V., Zhu, W., & Zeng, C. (2022). Artificial intelligence in early diagnosis and prevention of oral cancer. *Asia-Pacific Journal of Oncology Nursing, 9*(12), 100133.
26. Cai, Y., Xie, Y., Zhang, S., Wang, Y., Wang, Y., Chen, J., & Huang, Z. (2023). Prediction of postoperative recurrence of oral cancer by artificial intelligence model: Multilayer perceptron. *Head & Neck, 45*(12), 3053–3066.
27. Khanagar, S. B., Alkadi, L., Alghilan, M. A., Kalagi, S., Awawdeh, M., Bijai, L. K., et al. (2023). Application and performance of artificial intelligence (AI) in oral cancer diagnosis and prediction using histopathological images: A systematic review. *Biomedicine, 11*(6), 1612.
28. *The role of AI in cancer diagnosis and treatment: How technology is saving lives*. Retrieved May 2025, from https://mapmygenome.in/blogs/learn/the-role-of-ai-in-cancer-diagnosis-and-treatment-how-technology-is-saving-lives-1
29. Rajendran, S., Junaidi, N. D., Rajah, D. S., Nabil, A., Kipli, N., Maling, T. H., et al. (2025). Barriers and facilitators influencing the implementation of a mHealth (MeMoSA) oral cancer screening program in rural communities in a low-and middle-income country: Preliminary findings of a qualitative study. *Cancer Research, 85*(8_Supplement_1), 4900.
30. Morales-Gómez, C. B., Espinoza-Santander, I. L., López-Neira, L., von Marttens, A. H., Borgeat, M. C., Lee, X. M., et al. (2025). mHealth to enhance oral cancer awareness in older adults in Chile: A preliminary report. *Exploration of Digital Health Technologies, 3*, 101139.
31. Balasamy, S., Ganapathy, D., Nallaswamy, D., & Sundramoorthy, A. K. (2025). Uracil biomarker for pyrimidine metabolism in OSCC: Leveraging AI and machine learning for improved diagnosis. *The Open Dentistry Journal, 19*(1), e18742106360500.
32. Karuppan Perumal, M. K., Rajan Renuka, R., Kumar Subbiah, S., & Manickam Natarajan, P. (2025). Artificial intelligence-driven clinical decision support systems for early detection and precision therapy in oral cancer: A mini review. *Frontiers in Oral Health, 6*, 1592428.
33. Xu, Z., Lin, A., & Han, X. (2025). Current AI applications and challenges in oral pathology. *Oral, 5*(1), 2.
34. *Ethical challenges and limitations of AI in cancer treatment*. Retrieved May 2025, from https://vcarecancercenter.com/ethical-challenges-and-limitations-of-ai-in-cancer-treatment/

Chapter 4
Practical Demonstrations of AI for Oral Cancer Detection and Diagnosis

The theoretical underpinnings and methodological approaches for leveraging artificial intelligence in oral cancer management have been extensively discussed in preceding chapters. This chapter shifts the focus from "how" to "what" and "how well" these AI solutions perform in practical, real-world contexts. We present the implementation strategies, empirical results, and demonstrable impact of our multi-faceted AI framework designed for the early detection and diagnosis of oral cancer. By showcasing these practical applications, we aim to illustrate the tangible benefits and potential of AI in transforming clinical workflows and improving patient outcomes in oral oncology. This chapter synthesizes the findings from four key areas: risk stratification, RGB image classification, histopathology image classification, and a holistic analysis aid, demonstrating their integrated utility.

4.1 AI for Oral Cancer Risk Stratification

Effective early detection of oral cancer begins with identifying individuals at higher risk. This section demonstrates the implementation and performance of our AI-driven risk stratification model for oral cancer. This section presents a logistic regression-based model [1] for stratifying oral cancer (OC) risk using regularization and cross-validation techniques. Predictions are translated into clinical risk categories.

R. Thanki, S. Shah, *Artificial Intelligence for Early Detection and Diagnosis of Oral Cancer*, Signals and Communication Technology,
https://doi.org/10.1007/978-3-032-05056-4_4

4.1.1 Data Overview and Preprocessing

Oral squamous cell carcinoma (OSCC) represents the most common form of oral cancer and often arises from a background of modifiable risk factors such as smoking, alcohol consumption, and poor oral hygiene. Despite advances in treatment, survival rates remain suboptimal due to late-stage diagnosis in many regions [2]. The emergence of machine learning tools and data-driven decision-making in medicine has created a demand for large, annotated datasets that capture the multifactorial nature of cancer incidence and outcomes. The Oral Cancer Prediction Dataset [2, 3] responds to this need by offering a structured, multi-attribute dataset suitable for both traditional epidemiological analysis and machine learning model development. This dataset comprises over 85k patient records with variables spanning four major domains:

- **Demographic and Behavioral Factors**: Age, gender, tobacco use (smoked/chewed), alcohol consumption, dietary patterns, and family history of cancer.
- **Symptomatology and Clinical Presentation**: Presence of ulcers, white/red patches, difficulty swallowing, and anatomical tumor location.
- **Cancer Staging and Medical Information**: TNM staging, histopathology, diagnosis date, and treatment status.
- **Survival and Follow-up Data**: Time to recurrence, survival status, and duration of medical follow-up.

The implementation begins with loading the oral cancer prediction dataset. A critical step is the conversion of categorical features into a numerical format using one-hot encoding. This process creates binary columns for each unique category, ensuring that nominal data can be effectively used by the machine learning model. For instance, a "Gender" column with "Male" and "Female" would become two new columns, "Gender_Male" and "Gender_Female," with binary values (0 or 1). The target variable, "Oral Cancer (Diagnosis)," which is originally categorical ("No" or "Yes"), is transformed into numerical values (0 for "No" and 1 for "Yes"). This binary encoding is essential for compatibility with binary classification algorithms.

Numerical features undergo standardization using "StandardScaler." This technique scales features to have a mean of 0 and a standard deviation of 1. Standardization is crucial for algorithms sensitive to feature scales, like logistic regression, as it prevents features with larger numerical ranges from dominating the learning process. Finally, the preprocessed dataset is split into training (80%) and validation (20%) sets. A stratified split is employed (using "stratify = y") to ensure that the proportion of oral cancer cases (both "Yes" and "No") is maintained in both the training and testing sets. This prevents imbalanced class distribution from affecting model training and evaluation, leading to more reliable performance metrics.

4.1.2 Model Training

A logistic regression model with fivefold cross-validation ("LogisticRegressionCV") was chosen for this classification task. Logistic regression is a powerful and interpretable linear model commonly used for binary classification. Key parameters used in model training include:

- **cv = 5:** Specifies fivefold cross-validation. This technique divides the training data into five subsets; the model is trained on four subsets and validated on the remaining one, repeating this process five times. This helps in obtaining a more robust estimate of model performance and reduces the risk of overfitting.
- **penalty = l2:** Applies L2 regularization (Ridge regularization). L2 regularization adds a penalty equal to the square of the magnitude of coefficients to the loss function. This helps in shrinking the coefficients toward zero, preventing overfitting by reducing the model's complexity and making it more generalizable.
- **solver = liblinear:** An efficient solver for small datasets and L1/L2 regularization. It is well suited for binary classification problems.
- **scoring = roc_auc:** The model's performance during cross-validation is optimized based on the Area Under the Receiver Operating Characteristic Curve (AUC-ROC). AUC is a robust metric for imbalanced datasets, as it measures the model's ability to distinguish between positive and negative classes across all possible classification thresholds.
- **max_iter = 1000:** Sets the maximum number of iterations for the solver to converge. This ensures that the optimization algorithm has enough steps to find the optimal model parameters.

The trained logistic regression model, the "StandardScaler" object used for feature scaling, and the list of feature column names (after one-hot encoding) have all been saved to the "Trained Model/directory." This allows for easy reloading of the model and consistent preprocessing of new data for future predictions and deployments.

4.1.3 Risk Categorization

The model's predicted probabilities are translated into distinct clinical risk categories to provide actionable insights. The categorization is defined as follows:

- **Very Low Risk:** Predicted probability <0.1.
- **Low Risk:** $0.1 \leq$ Predicted probability <0.3.
- **Moderate Risk:** $0.3 \leq$ Predicted probability <0.6.
- **High Risk:** $0.6 \leq$ Predicted probability <0.9.
- **Very High Risk:** Predicted probability ≥ 0.9.

This stratification helps in a more intuitive understanding of a patient's risk profile and can guide further medical investigations or preventative measures.

4.1.4 Training Performance Evaluation

This section presents the model's performance on the training dataset. These metrics reflect how well the model has learned from the data it was trained on.

- **Training Confusion Matrix:** The Confusion Matrix (as shown in Fig. 4.1) for the training set shows the counts of True Positives (correctly predicted "Yes" cases), True Negatives (correctly predicted "No" cases), False Positives (incorrectly predicted "Yes" cases), and False Negatives (incorrectly predicted "No" cases) on the data the model was trained on. A high number of correctly classified instances here indicate effective learning.
- **Training ROC Curve:** The ROC curve (as shown in Fig. 4.2) for the training set illustrates the model's ability to discriminate between positive and negative classes across various thresholds. The Area Under the Curve (AUC) for the training set is 1.00. A high training AUC suggests that the model has learned to separate the classes well within the training data.
- **Training Risk Category Distribution:** Fig. 4.3 displays the distribution of predicted risk categories ("Very Low," "Low," "Moderate," "High," "Very High

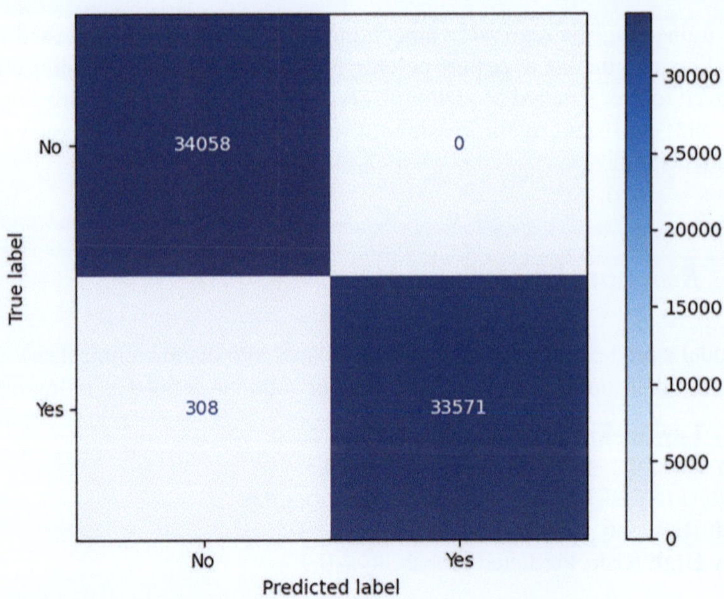

Fig. 4.1 Confusion matrix for training dataset

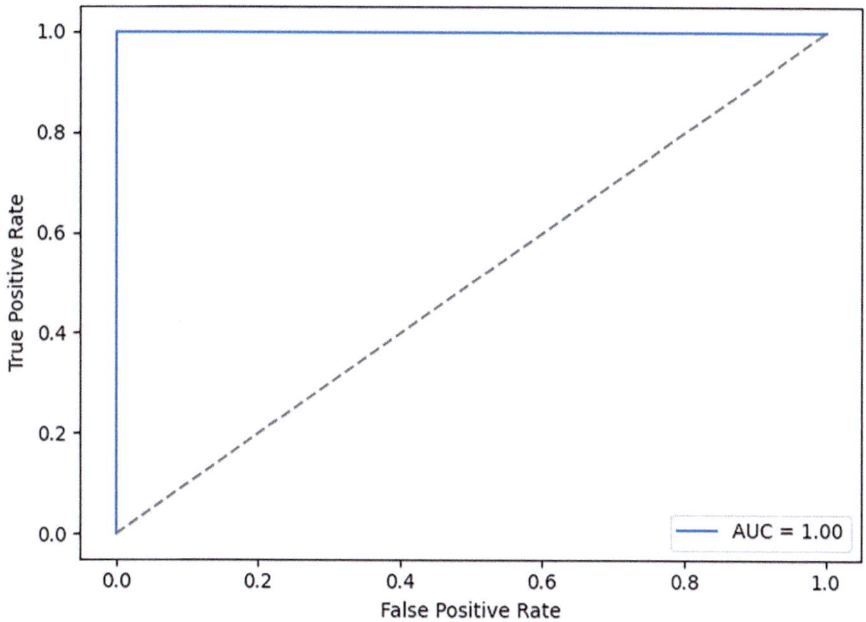

Fig. 4.2 ROC curve for training dataset

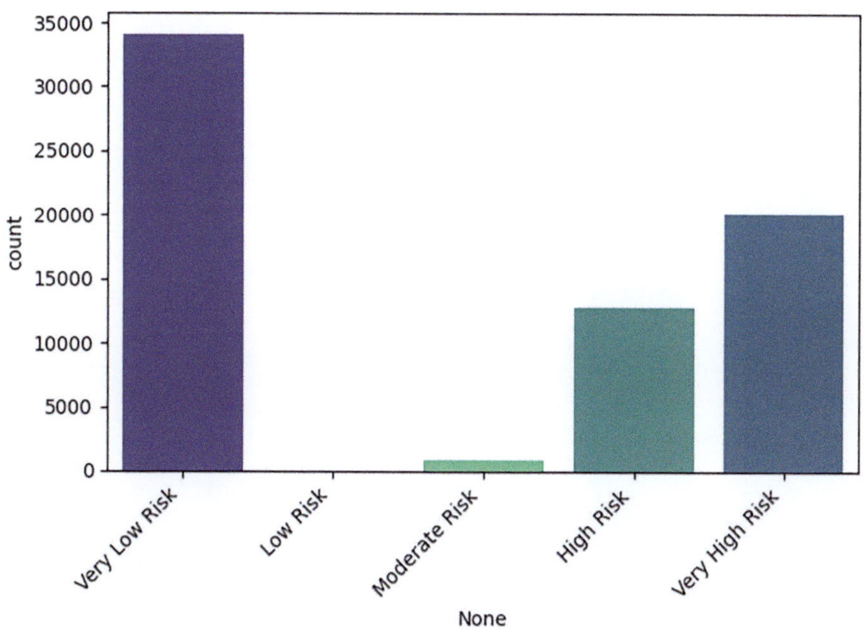

Fig. 4.3 Predicted risk category distribution for training dataset

Risk") on the training data. It helps in understanding how the model assigns risk levels to the data it has seen during training.

- **Training SHAP Interpretability:** SHAP values are calculated on the training dataset to understand how features contributed to the model's predictions during the learning phase. This provides insights into the relationships the model learned. The SHAP bar plot (as shown in Fig. 4.4) for the training dataset shows the average absolute impact of each feature on the model output. This provides a global view of feature importance during training. The SHAP beeswarm plot (as shown in Fig. 4.5) for the training set visualizes the distribution of SHAP values for each feature, indicating both the magnitude and direction of their impact on

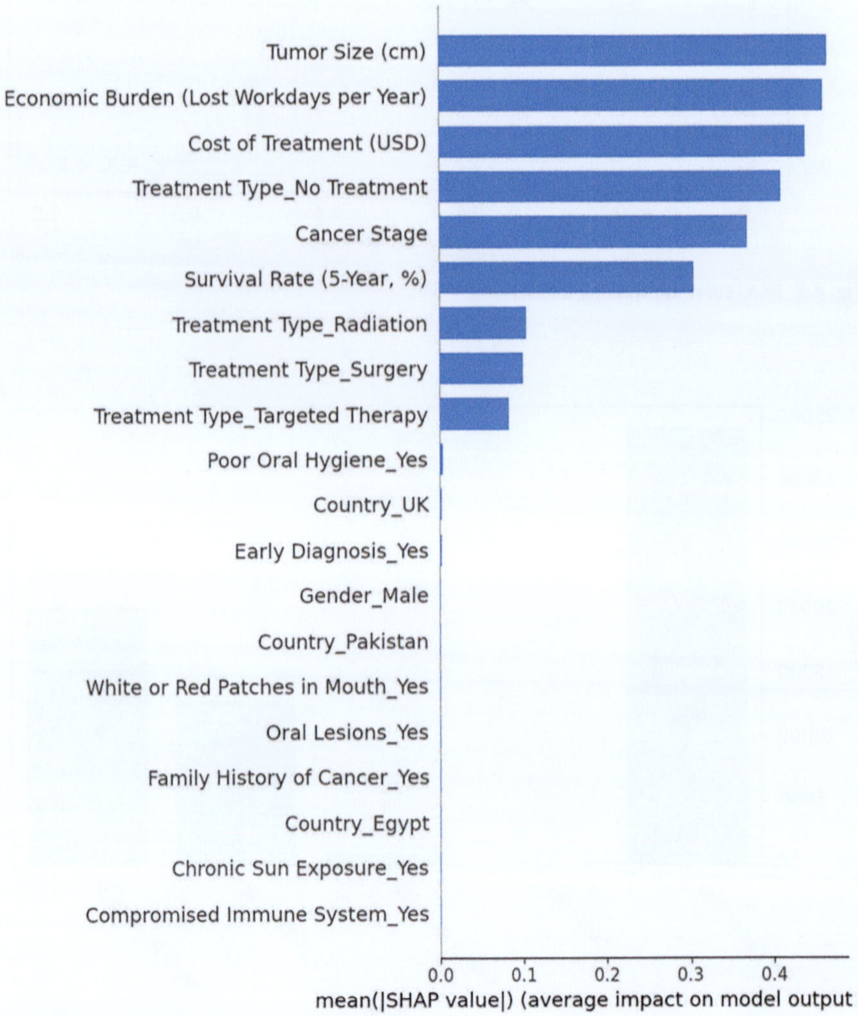

Fig. 4.4 SHAP values for training dataset

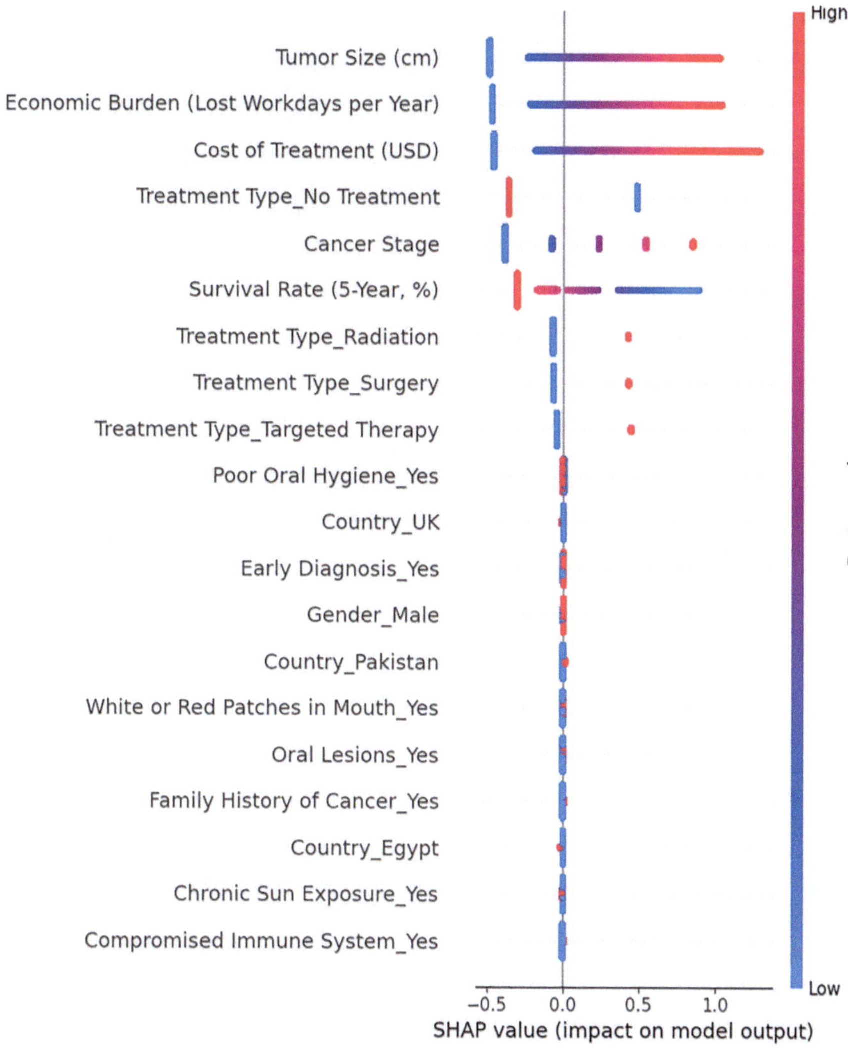

Fig. 4.5 SHAP beeswarm plot for training dataset

individual predictions within the training data. The color indicates the feature value (e.g., red for high, blue for low), helping to understand how different feature values influence predictions during training.

- **Training Classification Report:** The performance of the proposed model for training dataset was evaluated using standard classification metrics including precision, recall, F1-score, and accuracy, with results summarized in Table 4.1. These metrics provide a comprehensive understanding of the model's effectiveness across both classes: *No* and *Yes*.

The key observations from Table 4.1 are as follows:

Table 4.1 Classification performance metrics of training dataset for logistic regression (LR) model

Metrics	Precision	Recall	Fl-score	Support
No	0.99	1.00	1.00	34,058
Yes	1.00	0.99	1.00	33,879
Accuracy	1.00			67,937
Macro avg	1.00	1.00	1.00	67,937
Weighted avg	1.00	1.00	1.00	67,937

1. **High Overall Accuracy**: The model achieved an overall accuracy of 1.00, indicating that all predictions on the test dataset were correct. This demonstrates a highly reliable classifier.
2. **Class-wise Performance**:
    - For the "No" class:
        - **Precision**: 0.99—Only 1% of predicted "No" instances were incorrect.
        - **Recall**: 1.00—The model correctly identified all actual "No" instances.
        - **F1-score**: 1.00—The balance between precision and recall is excellent.
    - For the "Yes" class:
        - **Precision**: 1.00—All predicted "Yes" instances were correct.
        - **Recall**: 0.99—The model missed a very small fraction of actual "Yes" instances.
        - **F1-score**: 1.00—Again, a strong indicator of balanced classification.
3. **Support Values**: The dataset used for evaluation included 34,058 samples of class "No" and 33,879 samples of class "Yes," ensuring near-equal class distribution.
4. **Macro and Weighted Averages**: Macro average (unweighted mean of scores across both classes) and weighted average (weighted by support) for all metrics were 1.00. This reflects the model's consistency and robustness across both balanced and imbalanced scenarios.

These results suggest that the model generalizes well and maintains high predictive performance across both positive and negative classes. The marginal drop in recall for the "Yes" class could be a result of minor false negatives, which may be investigated further. Nonetheless, the metrics confirm that the model is highly suitable for real-world applications requiring high precision and recall such as in medical diagnostics or critical decision-making systems.

4.1.5 Validation Performance Evaluation

This section presents the model's performance on the unseen validation dataset. These metrics are crucial for assessing the model's generalization capability and its expected performance on new, real-world data.

- **Validation Confusion Matrix:** The confusion matrix (as shown in Fig. 4.6) for the testing set reflects the model's performance on unseen data. It is vital to observe if the model maintains its predictive accuracy on data, it has not been trained on. Discrepancies between training and testing confusion matrices might indicate overfitting.
- **Validation ROC Curve:** The ROC curve (as shown in Fig. 4.7) for the testing set is a key indicator of the model's ability to distinguish between positive and negative cases on new data. The Area Under the Curve (AUC) for the testing set is 1.00. A high testing AUC, like the training AUC, suggests good generalization and robustness of the model.
- **Validation Risk Category Distribution:** Fig. 4.8 shows the distribution of predicted risk categories ("Very Low," "Low," "Moderate," "High," "Very High

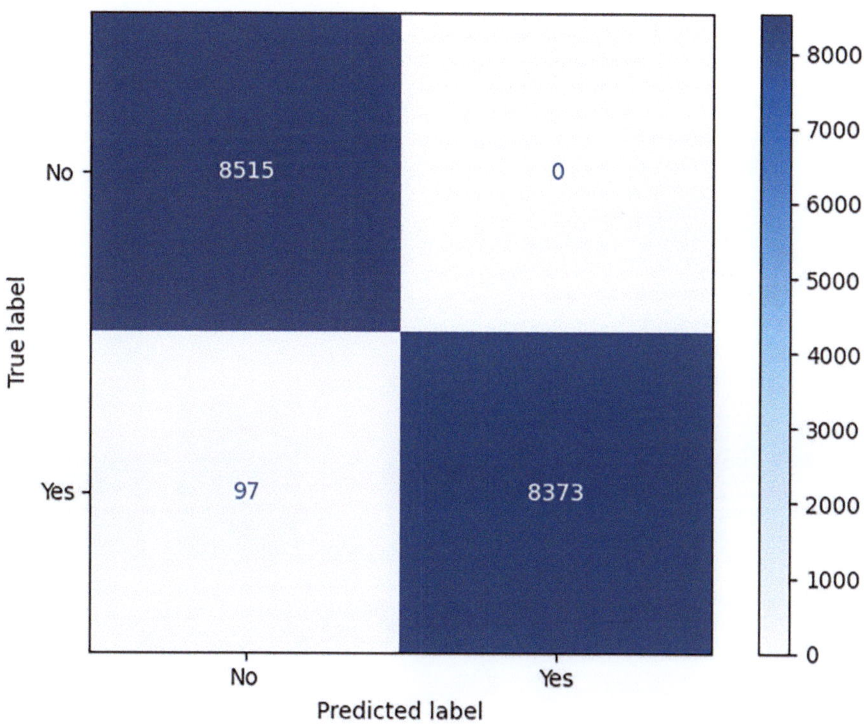

Fig. 4.6 Confusion matrix for validation dataset

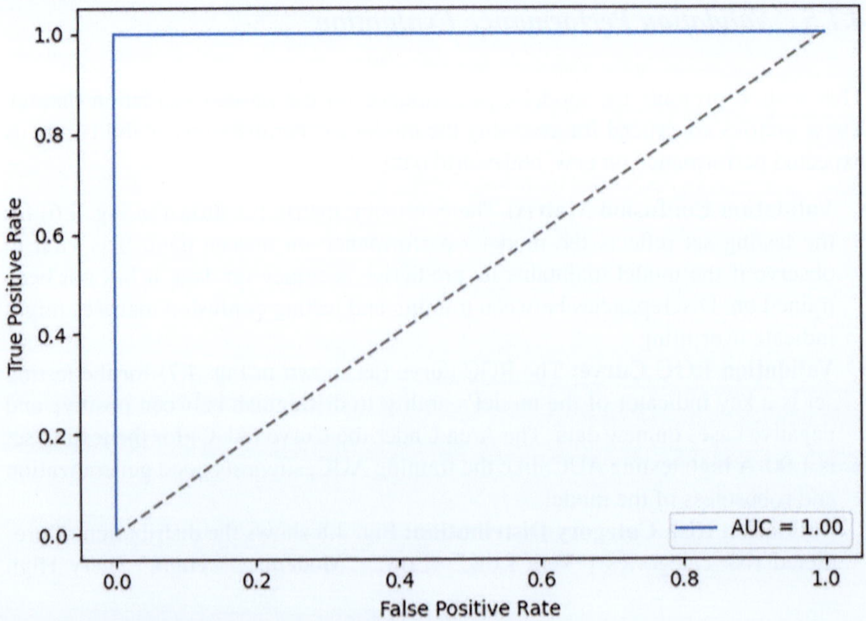

Fig. 4.7 ROC curve for validation dataset

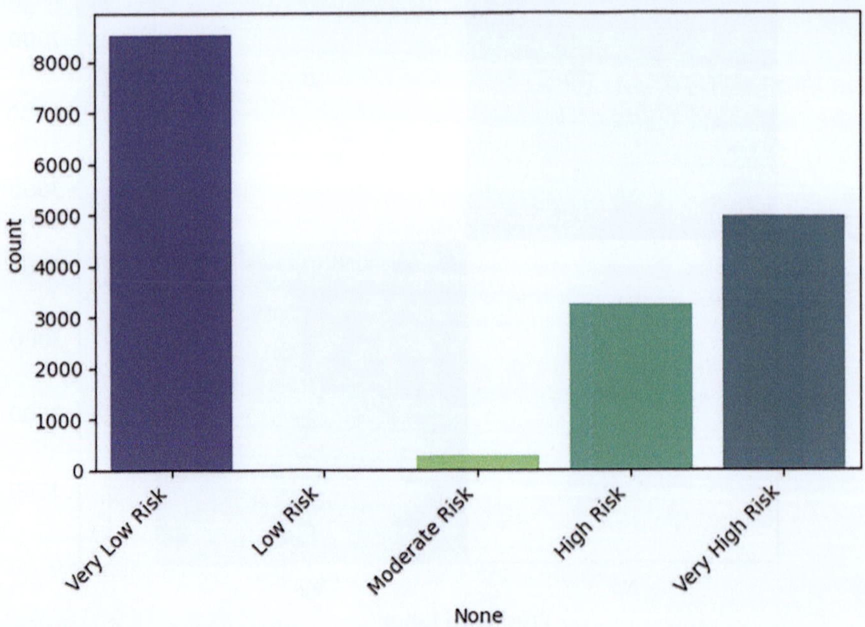

Fig. 4.8 Risk category distribution for validation dataset

Risk") on the unseen validation data. It indicates how the model stratifies risk for new patients.

- **Validation SHAP Interpretability:** SHAP values are calculated on the validation data to understand the contribution of features to predictions for unseen instances. This helps confirm whether the learned feature importance generalizes to new data. The SHAP bar plot (as shown in Fig. 4.9) for the validation dataset shows the average absolute impact of each feature on the model output for the unseen data. This provides a global view of feature importance on new instances. The SHAP beeswarm plot (as shown in Fig. 4.10) for the validation dataset provides detailed insight into how individual feature values influence predictions for

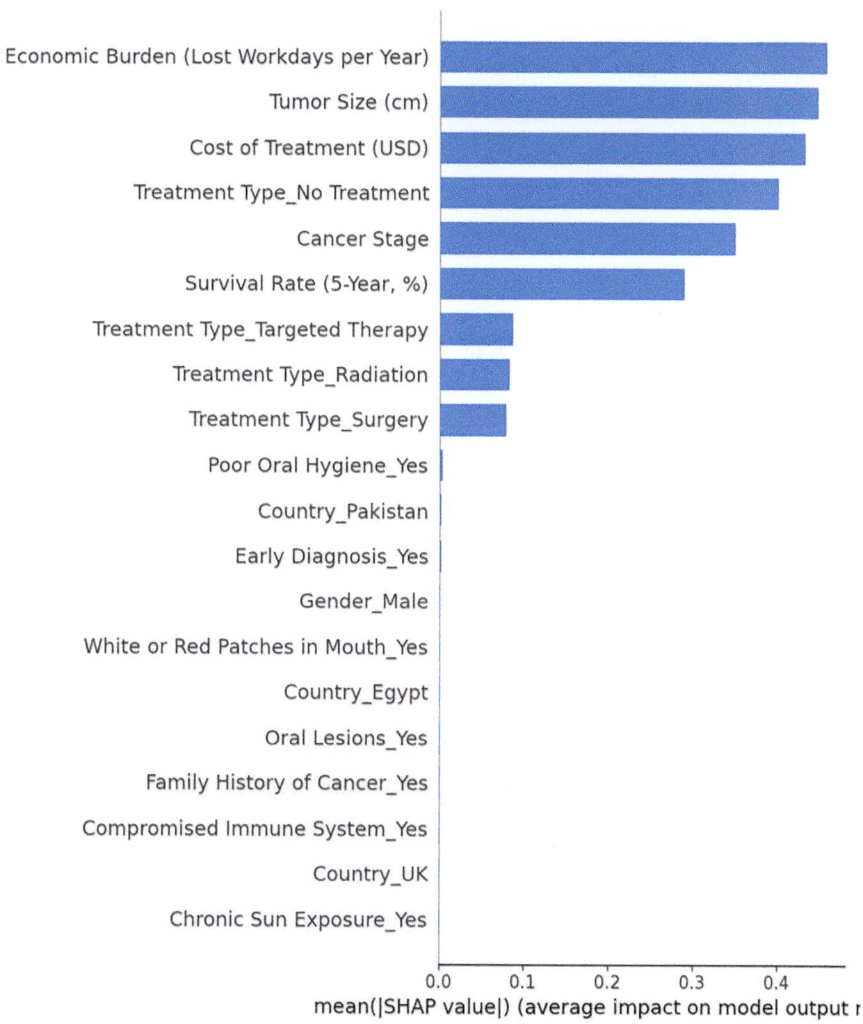

Fig. 4.9 SHAP values for validation dataset

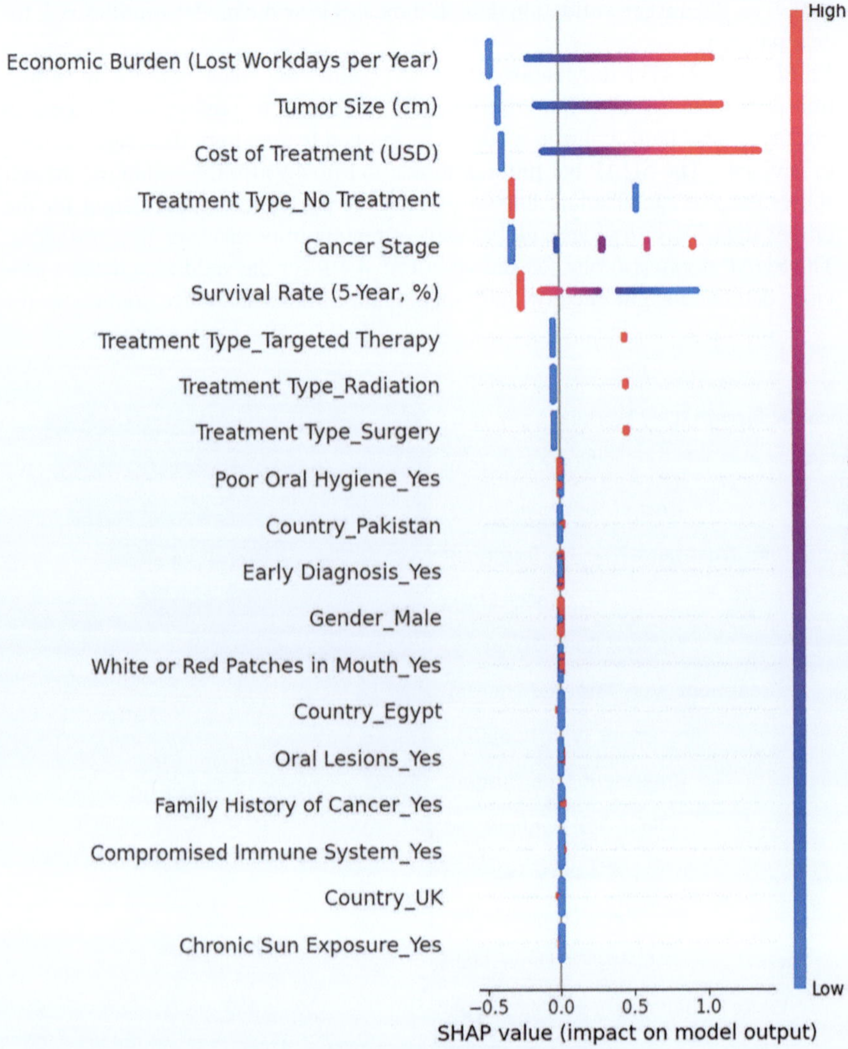

Fig. 4.10 SHAP beeswarm plot for validation dataset

unseen instances, revealing patterns of positive and negative contributions. Consistent patterns between training and validation SHAP plots suggest robust feature importance.

- **Validation Classification Report:** The performance of the proposed model for validation dataset was evaluated using standard classification metrics including precision, recall, F1-score, and accuracy, with results summarized in Table 4.2. These metrics provide a comprehensive understanding of the model's effectiveness across both classes: *No* and *Yes*.

The key observations from Table 4.2 are as follows:

Table 4.2 Classification performance metrics of validation dataset for logistic regression (LR) model

Metrics	Precision	Recall	Fl-score	Support
No	0.99	1.00	1.00	8515
Yes	1.00	0.99	0.99	8470
Accuracy	0.99			16,985
Macro avg	0.99	0.99	0.99	16,985
Weighted avg	0.99	0.99	0.99	16,985

1. **High Overall Accuracy**: The model achieved an overall accuracy of 0.99, indicating that 99% of predictions on the validation dataset were correct. This demonstrates that the classifier is highly reliable and capable of generalizing well to unseen data.
2. **Class-wise Performance**:
   - For the "No" class:
     - **Precision:** 0.99—Only 1% of predicted "No" instances were incorrect.
     - **Recall:** 1.00—The model correctly identified all actual "No" instances.
     - **F1-score:** 1.00—Indicates excellent balance between precision and recall, leading to highly accurate classification of the "No" class.
   - For the "Yes" class:
     - **Precision:** 1.00—All predicted "Yes" instances were correct.
     - **Recall:** 0.99—The model missed a very small fraction of actual "Yes" instances.
     - **F1-score:** 0.99—Strong performance, suggesting reliable detection of the "Yes" class.
3. **Support Values**: The validation dataset included 8515 samples labeled as "No" and 8470 samples labeled as "Yes,"indicating a balanced class distribution. This balance ensures that performance metrics are not skewed in favor of one class.
4. **Macro and Weighted Averages**: The macro average (unweighted mean across classes) for precision, recall, and F1-score is 0.99, showing that the model performs consistently well on both classes, independent of their size. The weighted average (weighted by class support) for all metrics is also 0.99, affirming that the model maintains excellent performance even when accounting for slight variations in class size.

These results confirm that the proposed model offers strong and balanced performance across all key metrics. Its ability to minimize both false positives and false negatives makes it a suitable candidate for deployment in critical applications such as medical diagnosis of oral cancer with risk level prediction.

4.1.6 Oral Cancer Risk Assessment Aid

The section gives the oral lesion AI risk assessment aid, a specialized application designed to provide a preliminary assessment of an individual's risk for oral lesions. Developed using advanced machine learning techniques, particularly a trained logistic regression (LR) model, this tool processes input data (e.g., patient information and associated oral imaging features) to generate a quantifiable risk prediction. The core objective is to offer an initial, data-driven indication of potential concern, assisting in early identification efforts. A visual representation of the application's user interface is provided in Fig. 4.11. showcasing its intuitive layout. It is paramount to understand that this AI-driven aid serves solely informational purposes and functions as a supplemental tool, not a replacement for professional medical diagnosis, comprehensive clinical evaluation, or treatment decisions.

The application streamlines the risk assessment process through its user-friendly interface, allowing healthcare professionals or trained personnel to easily input relevant patient data, typically via a structured CSV upload. Upon submission, the underlying CNN model analyzes the provided information to compute a probability score, which is then translated into a clear and actionable risk category (e.g., Very Low, Moderate, High Risk). This output is immediately presented within the application interface and can also be generated as a detailed HTML report, providing a comprehensive summary of the assessment, including patient input and the resulting risk level (as shown in Fig. 4.12b). This efficient and standardized approach to risk stratification aims to support clinical decision-making and facilitate timely referrals for further professional examination when a heightened risk is indicated.

It is imperative to note the inherent nature and limitations of this tool. As clearly stated within the application's interface, the "Oral Cancer Risk Assessment Aid" is developed for advanced informational and research purposes only. It is explicitly not designed to be a diagnostic device and should NOT replace professional medical advice, comprehensive clinical evaluation, diagnostic procedures, or the invaluable judgment of qualified healthcare professionals. Its purpose is to serve as an

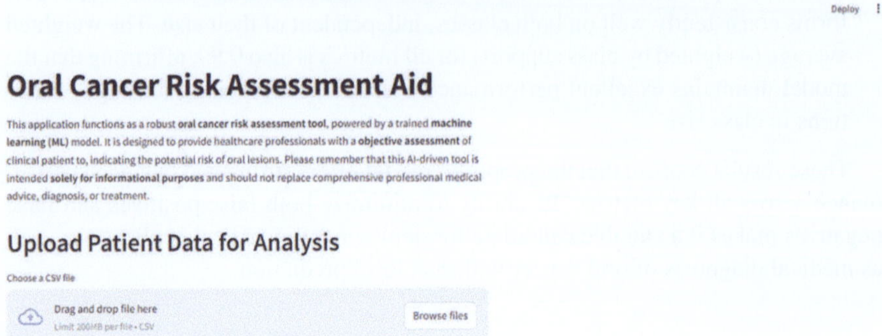

Fig. 4.11 UI of oral cancer risk assessment aid

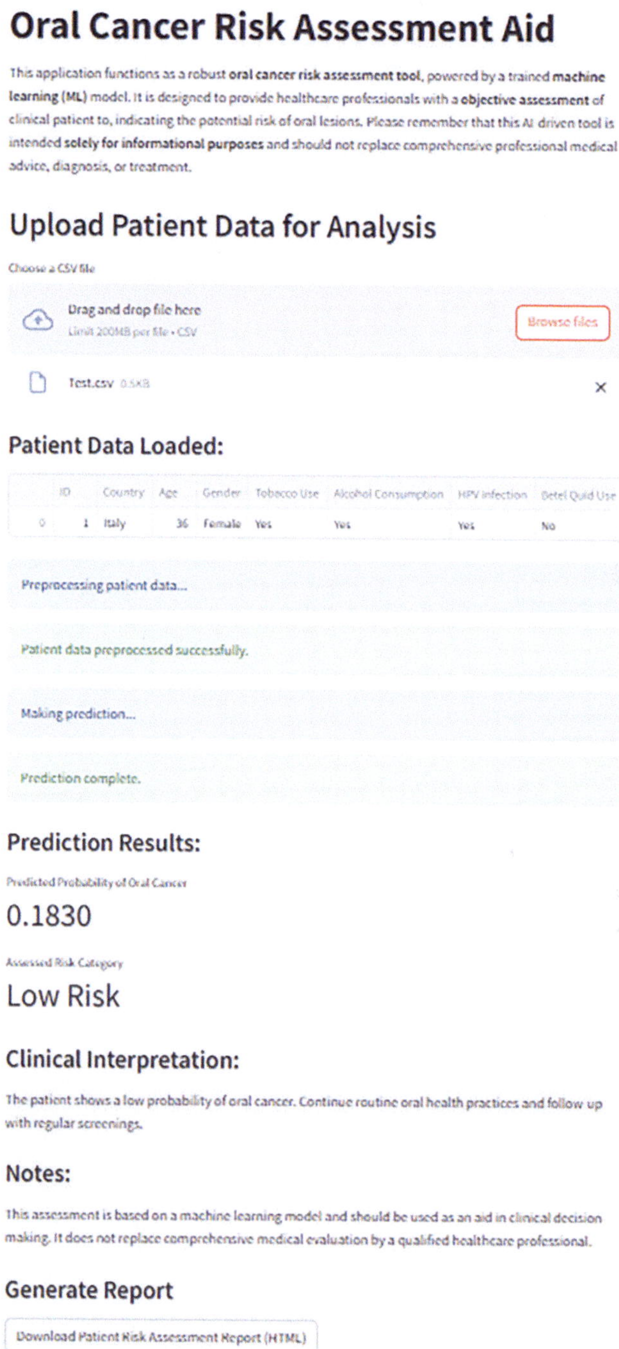

(a)

Fig. 4.12 Results generated by oral cancer risk assessment aid (**a**) after upload data and (**b**) detailed HTML report

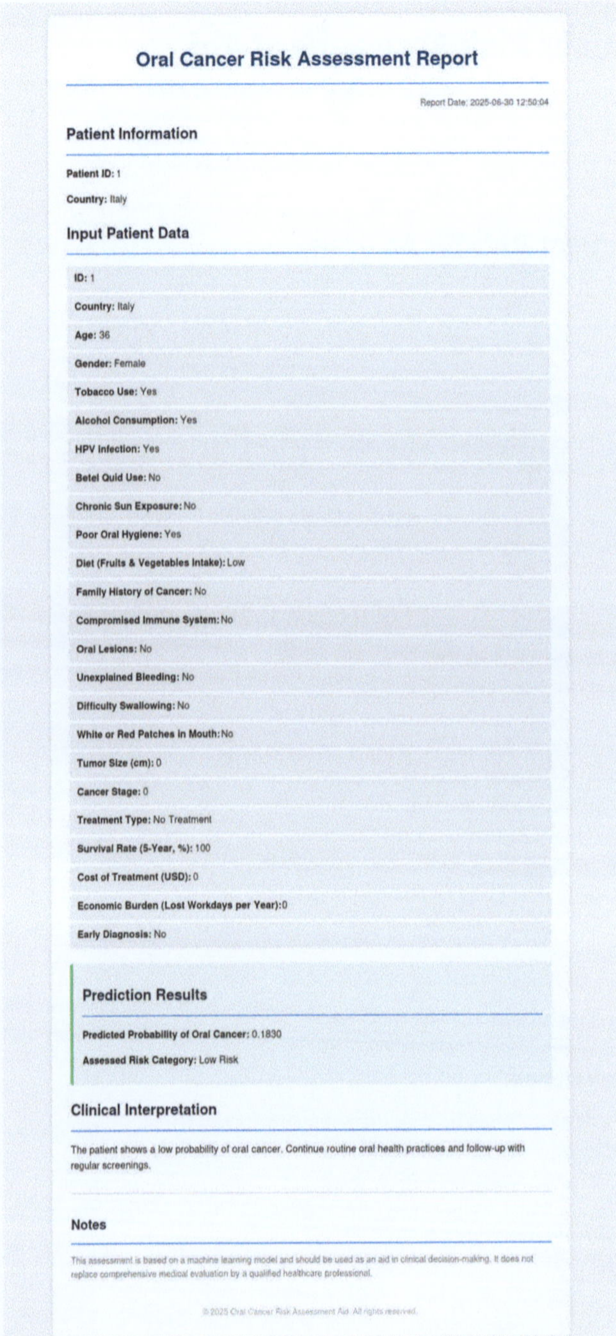

Oral Cancer Risk Assessment Report

Report Date: 2025-06-30 12:50:04

Patient Information

Patient ID: 1

Country: Italy

Input Patient Data

ID: 1

Country: Italy

Age: 36

Gender: Female

Tobacco Use: Yes

Alcohol Consumption: Yes

HPV Infection: Yes

Betel Quid Use: No

Chronic Sun Exposure: No

Poor Oral Hygiene: Yes

Diet (Fruits & Vegetables Intake): Low

Family History of Cancer: No

Compromised Immune System: No

Oral Lesions: No

Unexplained Bleeding: No

Difficulty Swallowing: No

White or Red Patches in Mouth: No

Tumor Size (cm): 0

Cancer Stage: 0

Treatment Type: No Treatment

Survival Rate (5-Year, %): 100

Cost of Treatment (USD): 0

Economic Burden (Lost Workdays per Year): 0

Early Diagnosis: No

Prediction Results

Predicted Probability of Oral Cancer: 0.1830

Assessed Risk Category: Low Risk

Clinical Interpretation

The patient shows a low probability of oral cancer. Continue routine oral health practices and follow-up with regular screenings.

Notes

This assessment is based on a machine learning model and should be used as an aid in clinical decision-making. It does not replace comprehensive medical evaluation by a qualified healthcare professional.

© 2025 Oral Cancer Risk Assessment Aid. All rights reserved.

(b)

Fig. 4.12 (continued)

intelligent assistant, augmenting human expertise in the complex domain of oral cancer assessment.

4.2 AI for Oral Cancer RGB Image Classification

This section provides a comprehensive overview of the training and evaluation performance of a Simple Convolutional Neural Network (CNN) model for binary classification of oral cancer RGB images. The goal is to classify images into distinct categories based on visual features. This section includes key training parameters, model architecture details, and various performance metrics to assess the model's effectiveness.

4.2.1 Dataset Information

The dataset [4] utilized in model development and evaluation comprises a total of 950 high-resolution oral cavity images, including 500 images of oral cancer cases and 450 images of non-cancerous oral tissues. Each image was carefully annotated and categorized to ensure clarity and consistency, making the dataset suitable for supervised machine learning applications in medical image analysis. The sample images of dataset are shown in Fig. 4.13.

To overcome the limitations posed by the relatively small number of original samples and to improve the robustness and generalizability of the classification model, data augmentation techniques were employed. Techniques such as rotation, flipping, zooming, and brightness adjustment were systematically applied to

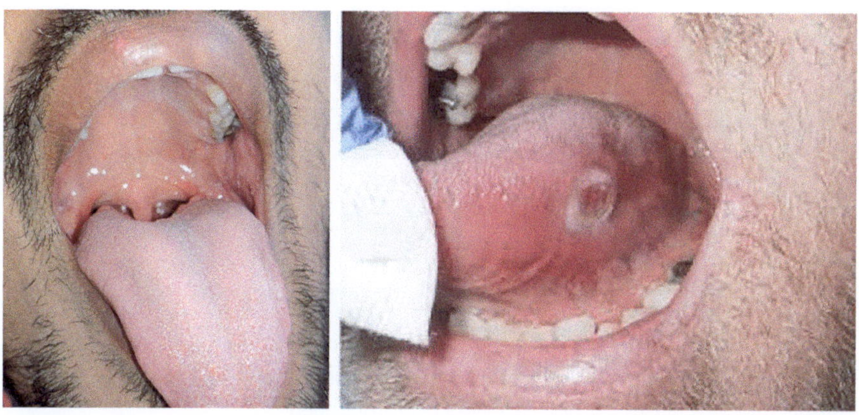

Fig. 4.13 Sample images of oral cavity image dataset

synthetically expand the dataset. As a result, the dataset was increased to 15,000 images, with a balanced representation of both cancerous and non-cancerous classes.

This augmented and balanced dataset provides a solid foundation for training deep learning models while reducing the risk of class imbalance and overfitting. It enables researchers to experiment with various architectures and algorithms aimed at enhancing diagnostic performance. Furthermore, the dataset supports broader objectives in the field of artificial intelligence-assisted medical diagnosis, especially in the context of early detection and intervention for oral cancer. Overall, this curated and expanded dataset represents a valuable resource for the research community, fostering innovation in the intersection of healthcare and machine learning. It serves as a stepping stone toward more accurate, accessible, and technology-driven solutions for oral cancer screening and diagnosis.

For the medical application, the class of this dataset label renamed as for "No Referral Needed" for non-cancerous cases and "Referral Warranted" for cancerous cases. The images were resized to a consistent dimension to fit the model's input requirements.

- Image dimensions used for processing: 224 × 224 pixels.
- Dataset divides into two sub datasets such as training dataset (80%) and validation dataset (20%).
- Batch size used during training: 32.
- Number of training epochs: 10.
- Identified class names: No referral needed, referral warranted.

4.2.2 *Model Architectures*

A SimpleCNN architecture built from scratch, designed to learn features directly from the image data. Table 4.3 provides a detailed summary of the model's layers, output shapes, and the number of parameters in each layer. This helps in understanding the complexity and structure of the neural network.

- Total params: 154,423,493 (589.08 MB).
- Trainable params: 51,474,497 (196.36 MB).
- Non-trainable params: 0 (0.00 B).
- Optimizer params: 102,948,996 (392.72 MB).

4.2.3 *Performance Details for SimpleCNN Model*

The following sections detail the performance of the SimpleCNN model on both the training and validation datasets after ten training epochs.

Table 4.3 Simple CNN model architecture

Model: "sequential"		
Layer (type)	Output shape	Param #
conv2d (Conv2D)	(None, 224, 224, 32)	896
max_pooling2d (MaxPooling2D)	(None, 112, 112, 32)	0
conv2d_1 (Conv2D)	(None, 112, 112, 64)	18,496
max_pooling2d_1 (MaxPooling2D)	(None, 56, 56, 64)	0
conv2d_2 (Conv2D)	(None, 56, 56, 128)	73,856
max_pooling2d_2 (MaxPooling2D)	(None, 28, 28, 128)	0
flatten (Flatten)	(None, 100,352)	0
dense (Dense)	(None, 512)	51,380,736
dropout (Dropout)	(None, 512)	0
dense_1 (Dense)	(None, 1)	513

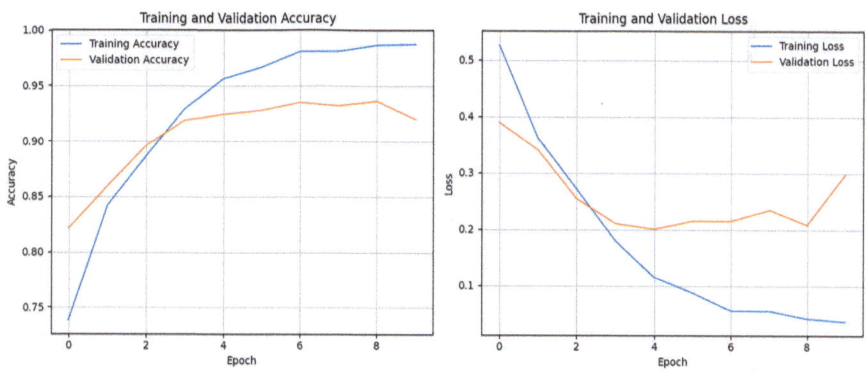

Fig. 4.14 Accuracy and loss plots for training and validation dataset

- **Training and Validation History:** The plot (as shown in Fig. 4.14) illustrates the SimpleCNN model's learning progress over the training epochs. The "Accuracy" plot shows how well the model performed on both the training and validation datasets over time, while the "Loss" plot indicates the error rate. Ideally, both training and validation metrics should improve and converge, without a significant gap indicating overfitting.
- **Model Performance Evaluation for Training Dataset:**

  The performance of SimpleCNN model evaluated using different metrics such as confusion, classification report, and ROC curve which are summarized in this section. The confusion metrics (as shown in Fig. 4.15) assess the SimpleCNN model's performance on the training dataset. While high performance here is expected, it's crucial to compare it with validation performance to detect overfitting.

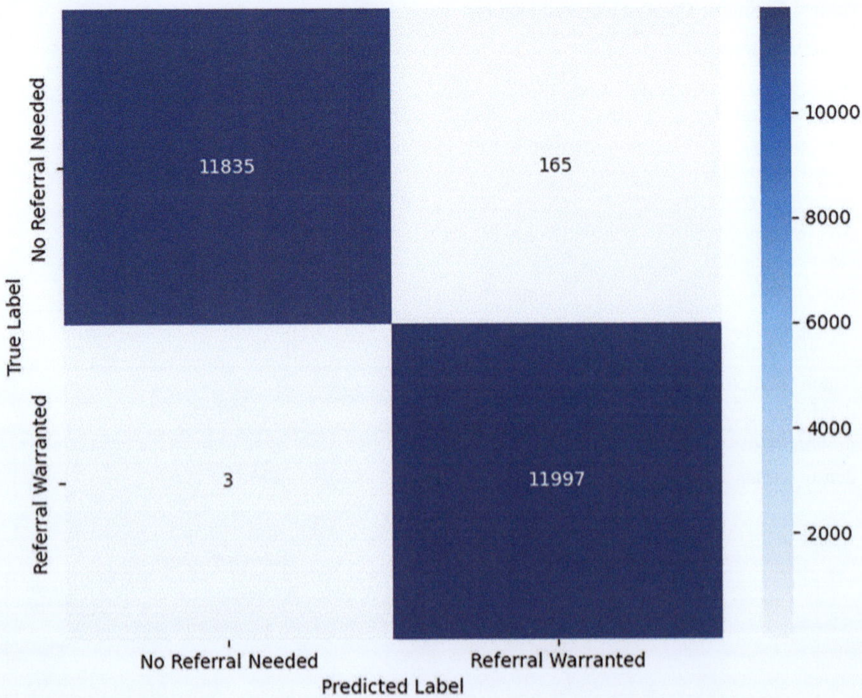

Fig. 4.15 Confusion matrix for training dataset

Table 4.4 Classification performance metrics of training dataset for SimpleCNN model

Metrics	Precision	Recall	Fl-score	Support
No referral needed	0.9997	0.9862	0.9930	12,000
Referral warranted	0.9864	0.9998	0.9930	12,000
Accuracy	0.9930			24,000
Macro avg	0.9931	0.9930	0.9930	24,000
Weighted avg	0.9931	0.9930	0.9930	24,000

The performance of the SimpleCNN model for training dataset was evaluated using standard classification metrics including precision, recall, F1-score, and accuracy, with results summarized in Table 4.4. These metrics provide a comprehensive understanding of the model's effectiveness across both classes: *no referral needed,* and *referral warranted.*

The key observations from Table 4.4 are as follows:

1. **High Overall Accuracy**: The SimpleCNN model achieved an overall accuracy of 0.9930, indicating that 99.30% of all predictions made on the training dataset were correct. This reflects the model's exceptional reliability and suitability for high-stakes applications, such as clinical decision-making in patient referral systems.

2. **Class-wise Performance**:
   - For the "No Referral Needed" class:
     - **Precision:** 0.9997—Nearly all instances predicted as "No Referral Needed" were accurate, with only a 0.03% false positive rate.
     - **Recall:** 0.9862—The model successfully identified 98.62% of actual "No Referral Needed" cases.
     - **F1-score:** 0.9930—This high score confirms excellent balance between precision and recall.
     - **Support:** 12,000—Indicates a large and well-represented portion of the dataset for this class.
   - For the "Referral Warranted" class:
     - **Precision:** 0.9864—About 1.36% of instances predicted as "Referral Warranted" were incorrect.
     - **Recall:** 0.9998—The model correctly detected 99.98% of actual "Referral Warranted" cases, minimizing false negatives a crucial factor in medical decision systems.
     - **F1-score:** 0.9930—High confidence in identifying at-risk cases with strong balance between false positives and false negatives.
     - **Support:** 12,000—Equal representation to the other class ensures balanced model training and evaluation.
3. **Macro and Weighted Averages**: The macro average (simple mean across classes) for precision, recall, and F1-score is 0.9931, confirming the model's balanced performance regardless of class frequency. Weighted average (accounting for class support) also yields 0.9930–0.9931 across all metrics, reaffirming consistent model effectiveness across the full dataset.

The ROC curve of SimpleCNN model for training dataset is shown in Fig. 4.16. This ROC curve indicates that the SimpleCNN model achieved perfect classification performance on its training data, with an AUC of 1.00. This means it was able to perfectly distinguish between the "no referral needed" and "referral warranted" classes it was trained on.

These results highlight the SimpleCNN model's robustness and reliability in classifying whether a patient needs a referral or not. The extremely high recall for the "Referral Warranted" class is particularly significant, as it indicates the model's strong potential to assist in early identification of critical cases, reducing the chances of missing patients who truly need further medical attention. Such performance makes this model highly suitable for deployment in clinical triage systems, telemedicine platforms, or screening programs where early intervention is crucial.

- **Model Performance Evaluation for Validation Dataset:**

  The performance evaluation of SimpleCNN model on this dataset will give how well this model will perform on unseen data and generalization ability in

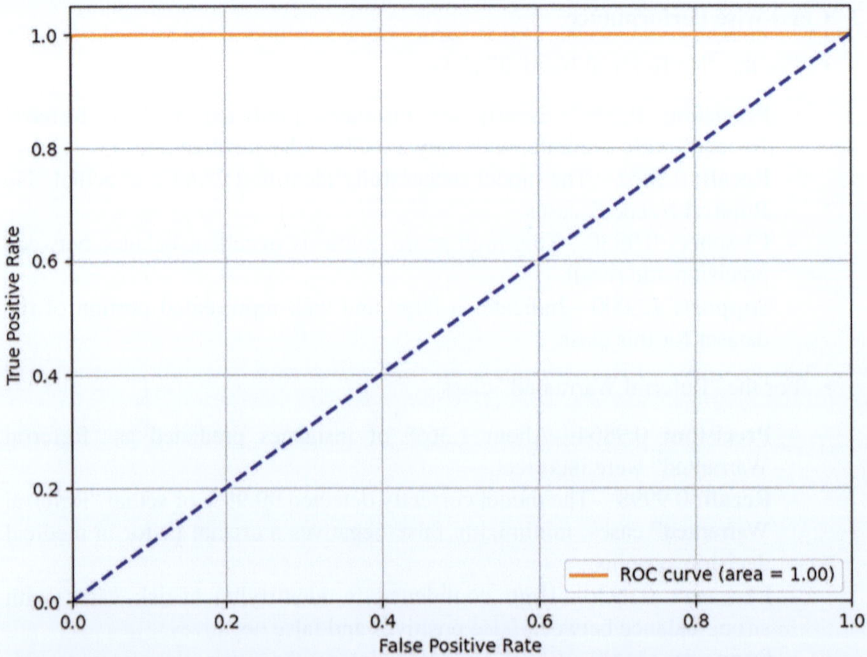

Fig. 4.16 ROC curve for training dataset

real-world scenarios. The confusion metrics (as shown in Fig. 4.17) assess the SimpleCNN model's performance on the validation dataset.

The performance of the SimpleCNN model for validation dataset was evaluated using standard classification metrics including precision, recall, F1-score, and accuracy, with results summarized in Table 4.5. These metrics provide a comprehensive understanding of the model's effectiveness across both classes: *no referral needed,* and *referral warranted*.

The key observations from Table 4.5 are as follows:

1. **High Overall Accuracy**: The SimpleCNN model achieved an overall accuracy of 0.9202 on the validation dataset, indicating that 92.02% of the predictions were correct. While not perfect, this performance is strong for a real-world binary classification task, especially in the healthcare domain where interpretability and early detection are prioritized.
2. **Class-wise Performance**:
    - For the "No Referral Needed" class:
        - **Precision:** 0.9762—The model was highly precise, with only 2.38% of predicted "No Referral Needed" instances being incorrect.

- **Recall: 0.8613**—The model successfully identified 86.13% of actual "No Referral Needed" cases, leaving room for improvement in detecting all true negatives.
- **F1-score: 0.9152**—This reflects a reasonably good balance between precision and recall, though slightly limited by the lower recall.
- **Support: 3000**—This class was equally represented in the dataset.

- For the "Referral Warranted" class:
  - **Precision:** 0.8759—About 12.41% of predictions for this class were false positives.

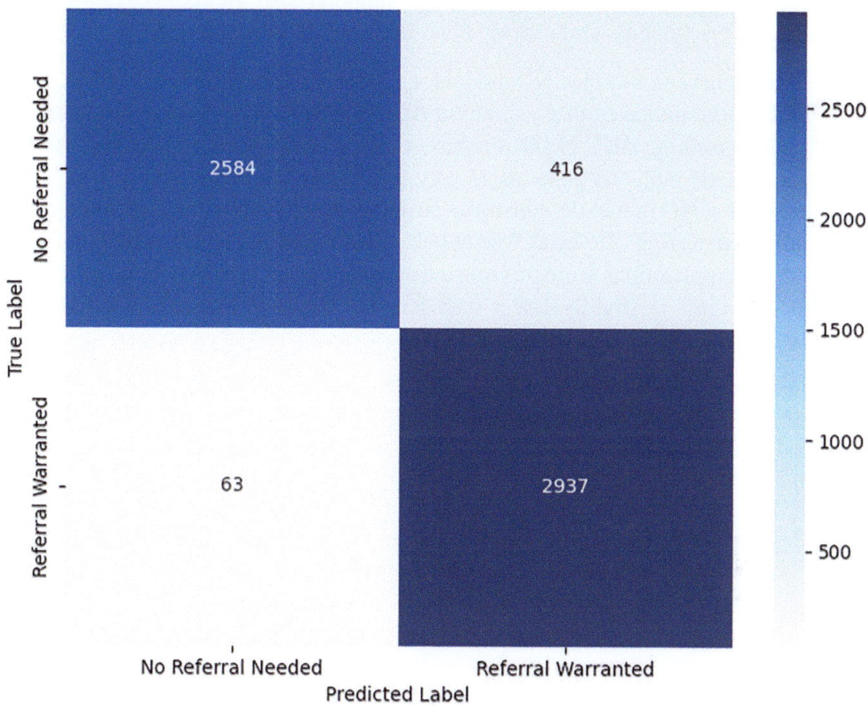

Fig. 4.17 Confusion matrix for validation dataset

Table 4.5 Classification performance metrics of validation dataset for SimpleCNN model

Metrics	Precision	Recall	Fl-score	Support
No referral needed	0.9762	0.8613	0.9152	3000
Referral warranted	0.8759	0.9790	0.9246	3000
Accuracy	0.9202			6000
Macro avg	0.9261	0.9202	0.9199	6000
Weighted avg	0.9261	0.9202	0.9199	6000

- **Recall:** 0.9790—The model successfully detected 97.90% of actual referral cases, minimizing false negatives, which is critical in clinical decision-making.
- **F1-score: 0.9246**—High score indicating effective identification of true positive referral cases.
- **Support: 3000**—Equal to the "No Referral Needed" class, maintaining class balance.

3. **Macro and Weighted Averages**: The macro average (simple mean across classes) for precision, recall, and F1-score is ~0.92, confirming the model's balanced performance across both classes without being biased by class size. Weighted average (accounting for class support) also yields ~0.9199–0.9261 across all predictions while taking class distribution into account.

The ROC curve of SimpleCNN model for validation dataset is shown in Fig. 4.18. This ROC curve indicates that validation AUC (0.98) is very close to, but slightly less than, the training AUC (1.00) suggests that the SimpleCNN model is performing exceptionally well and generalizes very effectively to unseen data.

The SimpleCNN model demonstrates strong generalization on the validation set, especially in detecting "Referral Warranted" cases with high recall, a critical factor in healthcare applications were missing a true positive can be risky. Although precision for this class is slightly lower than for "No Referral Needed," the trade-off

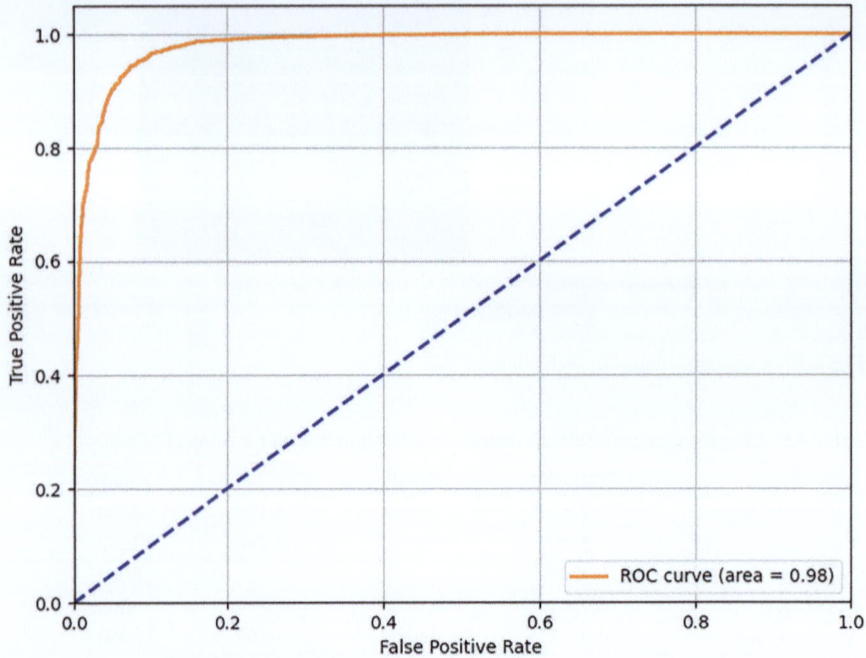

Fig. 4.18 ROC curve for validation dataset

favors sensitivity which is often desired in clinical triage systems. This performance highlights the SimpleCNN model's practical utility in decision support systems for medical referrals, with future improvements potentially focused on boosting recall for the "No Referral Needed" class without sacrificing overall accuracy.

4.2.4 *Oral Lesion AI Screening Aid*

This section introduces the Oral Lesion AI Screening Aid, a specialized application designed to assist in the preliminary assessment of oral images. Developed using the Streamlit framework for its user interface and leveraging various machine learning libraries in Python, this tool aims to provide an initial, informational screening for potential oral lesions. At its core, the application utilizes a sophisticated Convolutional Neural Network (SimpleCNN) model, which has been rigorously trained on a diverse dataset of oral images. This model is the engine behind the application's ability to analyze uploaded images and offer a prediction regarding the presence of anomalies. It's crucial to emphasize that this AI screening aid is intended solely for informational purposes and serves as a preliminary assessment tool, not a substitute for professional medical advice, diagnosis, or treatment. A screenshot of the application's user interface is provided in Fig. 4.19, illustrating its intuitive design.

The user experience of the oral lesion AI screening aid is designed to be intuitive and straightforward, facilitating easy interaction for healthcare professionals or individuals seeking an initial assessment. Users can effortlessly upload an oral image for analysis, either by dragging and dropping the file into the designated area or by utilizing the "Browse files" option. The application supports common image formats such as JPG, JPEG, PNG, and BMP, with a sensible size limit of 200 MB per file to ensure efficient processing. Once an image is submitted, the integrated

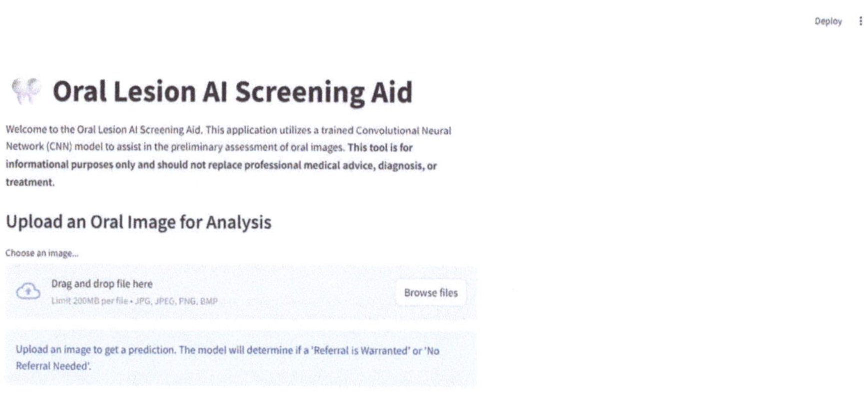

Fig. 4.19 UI of oral lesion AI screening aid

SimpleCNN model processes the visual data and provides a clear output: either "Referral is Warranted" or "No Referral Needed." Examples of the results generated by the application are depicted in Fig. 4.20a, b. This direct and actionable feedback streamlines the initial screening process, potentially aiding in identifying cases that may require further professional examination, thereby enhancing early detection efforts in oral health."

It is imperative to note the inherent nature and limitations of this tool. As clearly stated within the application's interface, the "Oral Lesion AI Screening Aid" is

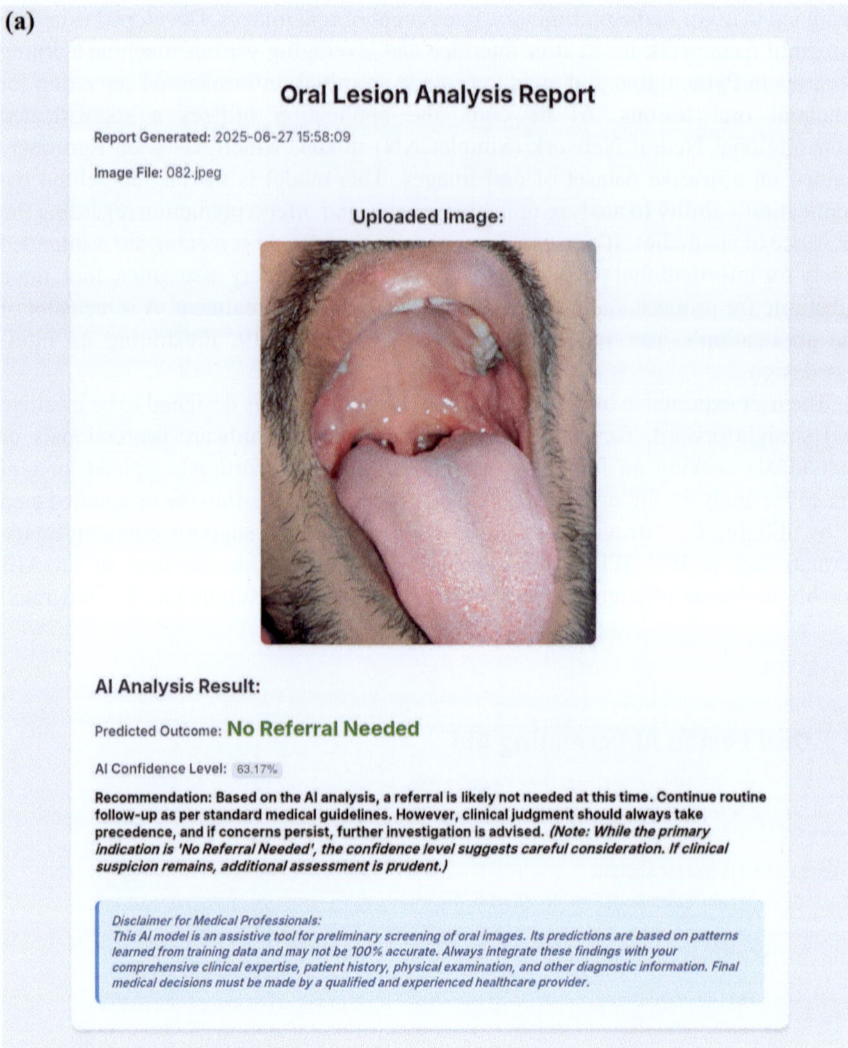

Fig. 4.20 Results generated by oral lesion AI screening aid (**a**) Case 1 and (**b**) Case 2

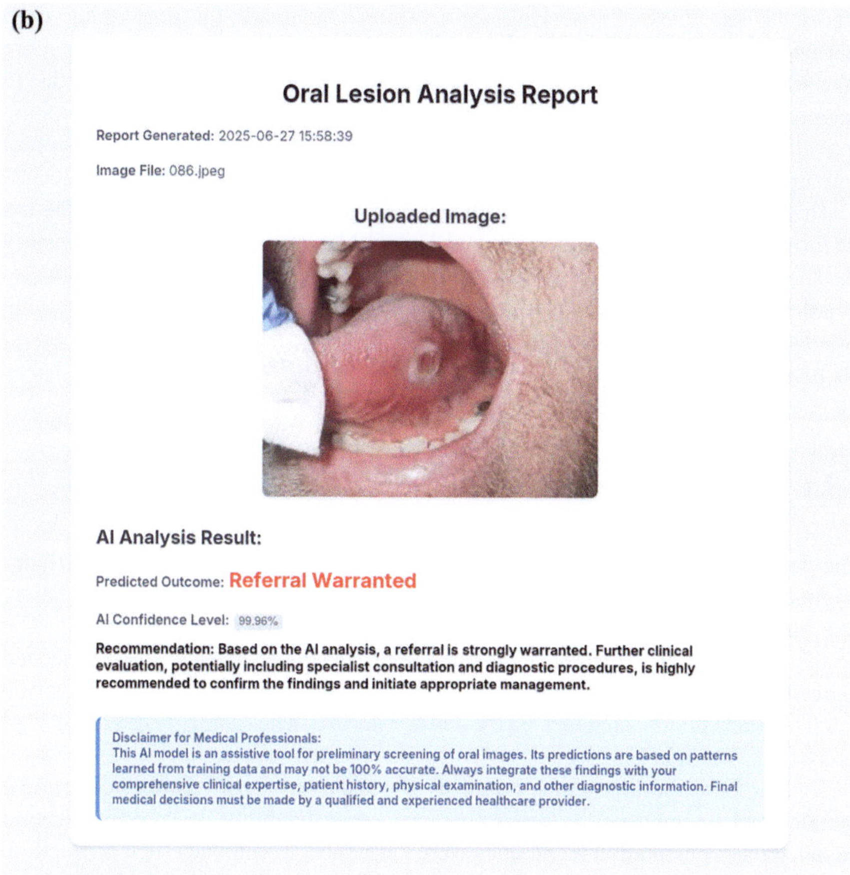

Fig. 4.20 (continued)

developed for advanced informational and research purposes only. It is explicitly not designed to be a diagnostic device and should NOT replace professional medical advice, comprehensive clinical evaluation, diagnostic procedures, or the invaluable judgment of qualified healthcare professionals. Its purpose is to serve as an intelligent assistant, augmenting human expertise in the complex domain of oral cancer assessment.

4.3 AI for Oral Cancer Histopathology Image Classification

Histopathological examination remains the gold standard for diagnosing oral squamous cell carcinoma (OSCC). The histopathologic oral cancer detection dataset is a curated collection of high-resolution histology patches, annotated with binary labels ("normal" vs. "OSCC"), serving as a prime benchmark for developing deep learning-based diagnostic systems in OSCC detection. OSCC accounts for more than 90% of all oral malignancies and is associated with significant mortality due to delayed detection. Automated image-based histopathology solutions leveraging convolutional neural networks (CNNs) have emerged as promising tools to support pathologists and reduce diagnostic variability and workload.

This section provides a comprehensive overview of the training and evaluation performance of a Simple Convolutional Neural Network (CNN) model for binary classification of oral cancer histopathology Images. The goal is to classify images into distinct categories based on visual features. This section includes key training parameters, model architecture details, and various performance metrics to assess the model's effectiveness.

4.3.1 Dataset Information

The dataset derived from Rahman et al. [5] and extended via Kaggle [6] includes original H & E-stained biopsy images captured at 100× and 400× magnification. The based dataset has 1224 images including 290 normal and 934 OSCC. The Kaggle expanded set with data augmentation up to 5192 samples; caution is needed to avoid leakage [7]. The binary class labels indicate where the central region of a patch contains OSCC such as 1 = sick and 0 = normal. The sample H & E images of dataset are shown in Fig. 4.21.

To overcome the limitations posed by the relatively small number of original samples and to improve the robustness and generalizability of the classification model, data augmentation techniques were employed. Techniques such as rotation, flipping, zooming, and brightness adjustment were systematically applied to synthetically expand the histopathology dataset. As a result, the dataset was increased to 15,000 images, with a balanced representation of both normal and OSCC classes.

This augmented and balanced dataset provides a solid foundation for training deep learning models while reducing the risk of class imbalance and overfitting. It enables researchers to experiment with various architectures and algorithms aimed at enhancing diagnostic performance. Furthermore, the dataset supports broader objectives in the field of artificial intelligence-assisted medical diagnosis, especially in the context of early detection and intervention for oral cancer. Overall, this curated and expanded dataset represents a valuable resource for the research community, fostering innovation in the intersection of healthcare and machine learning. It serves as a stepping stone toward more accurate, accessible, and technology-driven solutions for oral cancer screening and diagnosis. The images were resized to a consistent dimension to fit the model's input requirements.

- Image dimensions used for processing: 224 × 224 pixels.
- Dataset divides into two sub datasets such as training dataset (80%) and validation dataset (20%).

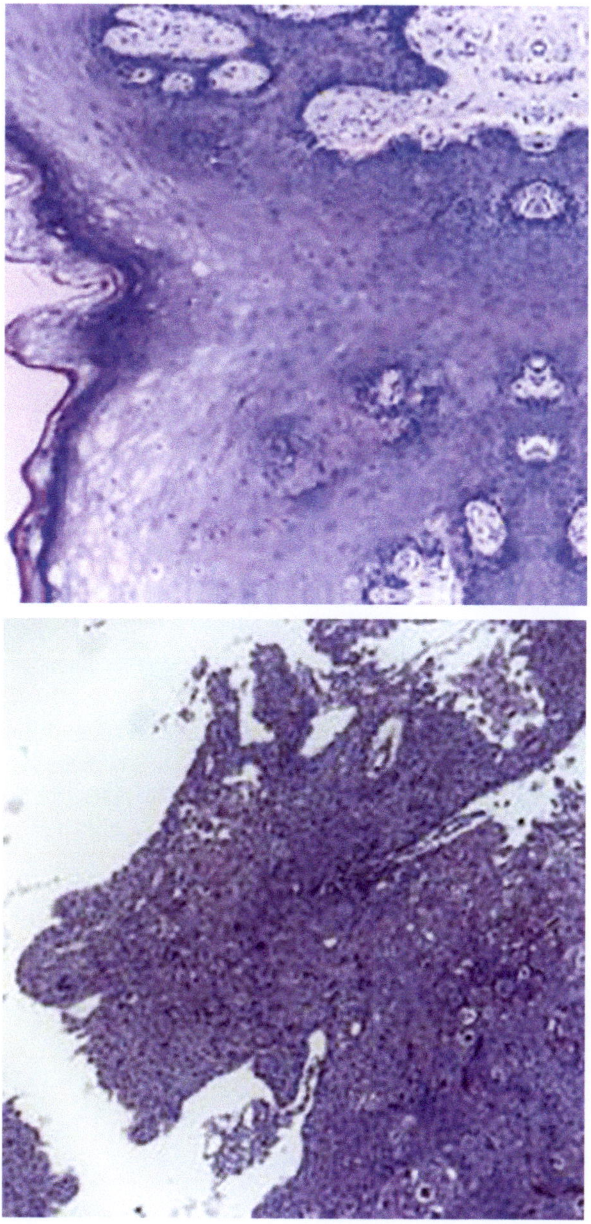

Fig. 4.21 Sample images of oral histopathology dataset

- Batch size used during training: 32.
- Number of training epochs: 10.
- Identified class names: Normal and OSCC.

4.3.2 Model Architectures

The same SimpleCNN architectures described in Sect. 4.2.2 are used in the histopathology oral cancer classification. The name of this trained model gives SimpleCNN_Histo to differentiate from the previous trained model.

4.3.3 Performance Details for SimpleCNN_Histo Model

The following sections detail the performance of the SimpleCNN_Histo model on both the training and validation datasets after ten training epochs.

- **Training and Validation History:** The plot (as shown in Fig. 4.22) illustrates the SimpleCNN_Histo model model's learning progress over the training epoch. The "Accuracy" plot shows how well the model performed on both the training and validation datasets over time, while the "Loss" plot indicates the error rate. Ideally, both training and validation metrics should improve and converge, without a significant gap indicating overfitting.
- **Model Performance Evaluation for Training Dataset:**

  The performance of SimpleCNN_Histo model evaluated using different metrics such as confusion, classification report, and ROC curve which are summarized in this section. The confusion metrics (as shown in Fig. 4.23) assess the SimpleCNN_Histo model's performance on the training dataset. While high performance here

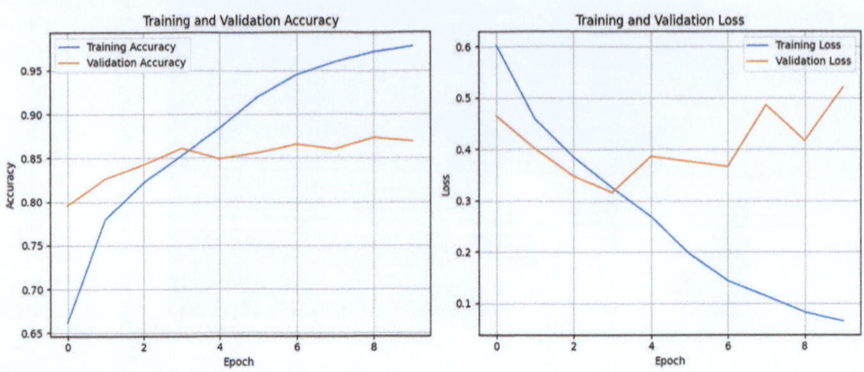

Fig. 4.22 Accuracy and loss plots for training and validation dataset

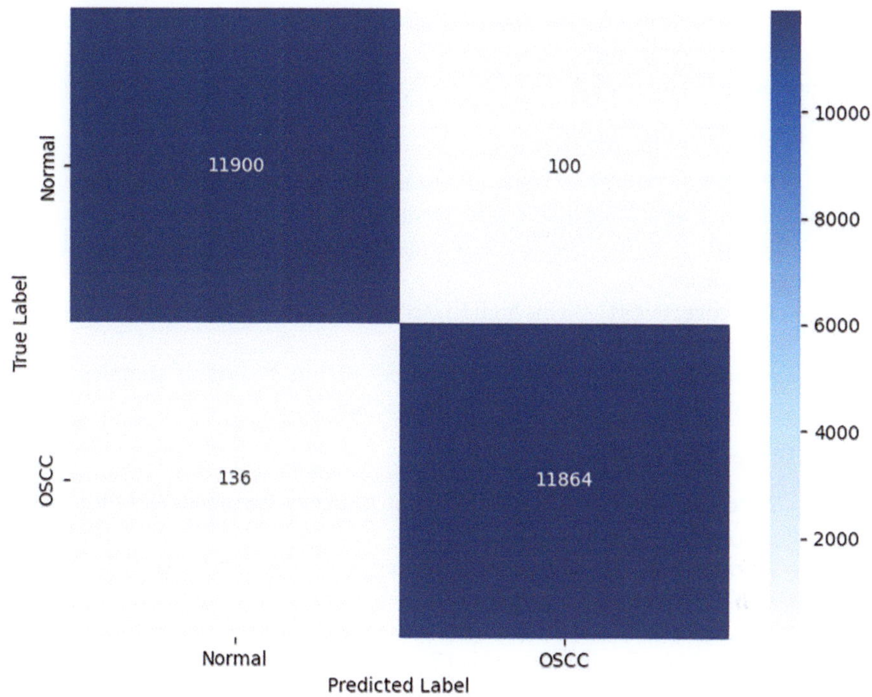

Fig. 4.23 Confusion matrix for training dataset

Table 4.6 Classification performance metrics of training dataset for SimpleCNN_Histo model

Metrics	Precision	Recall	Fl-score	Support
Normal	0.9987	0.9917	0.9902	12,000
OSCC	0.9916	0.9887	0.9902	12,000
Accuracy	0.9902			24,000
Macro avg	0.9902	0.9902	0.9902	24,000
Weighted avg	0.9902	0.9902	0.9902	24,000

is expected, it's crucial to compare it with validation performance to detect overfitting.
The performance of the SimpleCNN_Histo model for training dataset was evaluated using standard classification metrics including precision, recall, F1-score, and accuracy, with results summarized in Table 4.6. These metrics provide a comprehensive understanding of the model's effectiveness across both classes: *Normal,* and *OSCC*.

The key observations from Table 4.6 are as follows:

1. **High Overall Accuracy**: The SimpleCNN_Histo model achieved an accuracy of 0.9902 on the training dataset, indicating that 99.02% of predictions were correct. This high performance reflects the model's strong learning capacity on the

training data and its effectiveness in distinguishing between normal and cancerous (OSCC) oral images.

2. **Class-wise Performance**:

   - For the "Normal" class:

     – **Precision:** 0.9987—Nearly all instances predicted as "Normal" were truly normal, with a negligible false positive rate.
     – **Recall:** 0.9917—The model correctly identified 99.17% of actual normal cases.
     – **F1-score:** 0.9902—This high F1-score indicates excellent balance between precision and recall.
     – **Support:** 12,000—Shows the number of true "Normal" samples in the training set, ensuring balanced representation.

   - For the "OSCC" class:

     – **Precision:** 0.9916—About 0.84% of instances predicted as OSCC were incorrect.
     – **Recall:** 0.9887—The model successfully identified 98.87% of true OSCC cases.
     – **F1-score:** 0.9902—Strong agreement between precision and recall, confirming accurate identification of cancerous cases.
     – **Support:** 12,000—Equal to the "Normal" class, reinforcing dataset balance during training.

3. **Macro and Weighted Averages**: The macro average (simple mean across classes) for precision, recall, and F1-score is 0.9902, confirming the model's balanced performance regardless of class frequency. Weighted average (accounting for class support) also yields 0.9902 considering class distribution (equal here), reaffirming overall consistency.

The ROC curve of SimpleCNN_Histo model for training dataset is shown in Fig. 4.24. This ROC curve with an AUC of 1.00 signifies that the SimpleCNN_Histo model being evaluated achieves perfect discrimination between the two classes (e.g., Normal vs. OSCC). This means there's a threshold at which the model correctly identifies all positive cases and all negative cases, without any overlap or misclassification.

The results show that SimpleCNN_Histo as high-performing and well-generalized model, capable of accurately distinguishing between normal oral tissues and OSCC. The extremely high precision and recall for both classes suggest minimal misclassification and an effective learning process. Such results are promising for downstream applications in AI-assisted oral cancer screening, providing confidence in the model's ability to handle large-scale datasets.

- **Model Performance Evaluation for Validation Dataset:**
  The confusion metrics (as shown in Fig. 4.25) assess the SimpleCNN_Histo model's performance on the validation dataset.

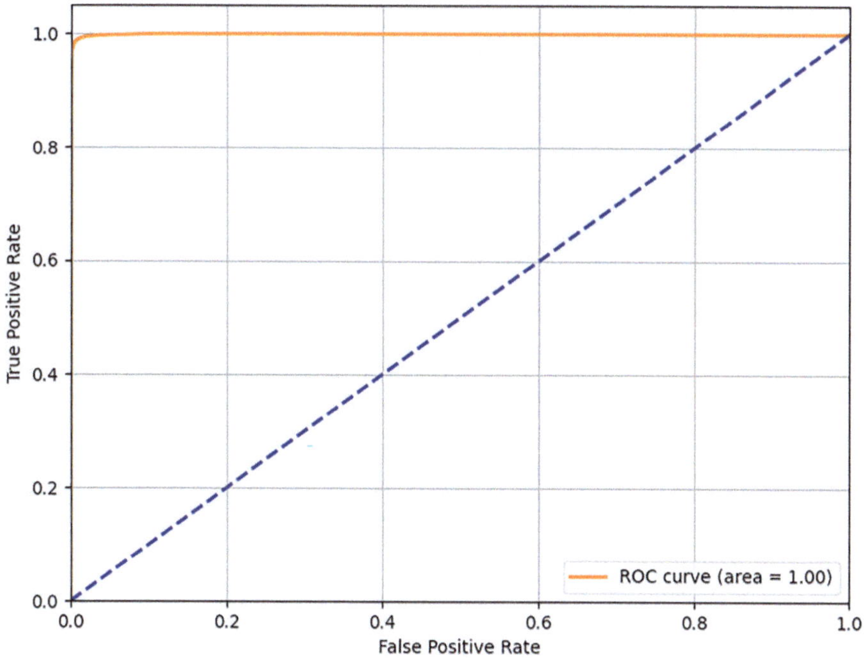

Fig. 4.24 ROC curve for training dataset

The performance of the SimpleCNN_Histo model for validation dataset was evaluated using standard classification metrics including precision, recall, F1-score, and accuracy, with results summarized in Table 4.7. These metrics provide a comprehensive understanding of the model's effectiveness across both classes: *Normal* and *OSCC*.

The key observations from Table 4.7 are as follows:

1. **High Overall Accuracy**: The SimpleCNN_Histo model achieved an overall accuracy of 0.8690 on the validation dataset, meaning that 86.90% of all predictions were correct. This suggests reasonable classification performance, with room for improvement, particularly in optimizing both sensitivity and specificity across classes.
2. **Class-wise Performance**:
    - For the "Normal" class:
        - **Precision:** 0.8815–88.15% of the samples predicted as "Normal" were truly normal, indicating a relatively low false positive rate.
        - **Recall:** 0.8527—The model correctly identified 85.27% of actual "Normal" cases, missing some true negatives.
        - **F1-score:** 0.8668—This reflects a fair balance between precision and recall for the "Normal" class.

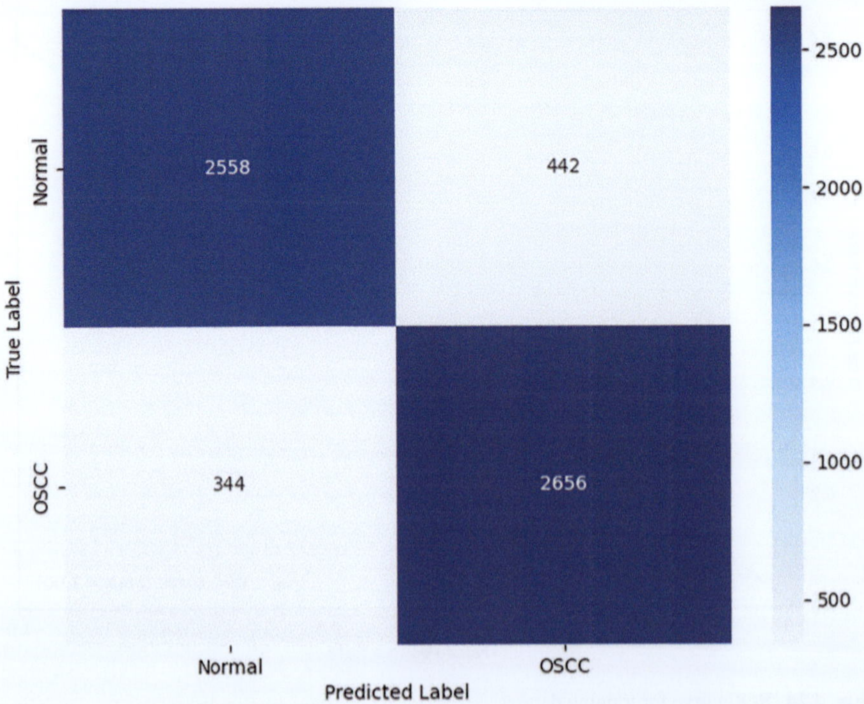

Fig. 4.25 Confusion matrix for validation dataset

Table 4.7 Classification performance metrics of validation dataset for SimpleCNN_Histo model

Metrics	Precision	Recall	Fl-score	Support
Normal	0.8815	0.8527	0.8668	3000
OSCC	0.8573	0.8853	0.8711	3000
Accuracy	0.8690			6000
Macro avg	0.8694	0.8690	0.8690	6000
Weighted avg	0.8694	0.8690	0.8690	6000

  – **Support:** 3000—Represents a well-distributed class within the validation dataset.

- For the "OSCC" class:
  – **Precision:** 0.8573—About 14.27% of predictions labeled as "OSCC" were incorrect.
  – **Recall:** 0.8853—The model identified 88.53% of actual OSCC cases, showing slightly better recall than the "Normal" class.
  – **F1-score:** 0.8711—Indicates reliable detection of OSCC instances with moderate class performance balance.
  – **Support:** 3000—Equal representation with the "Normal" class ensures fairness in evaluation.

3. **Macro and Weighted Averages**: The macro average (simple mean across classes) for precision, recall, F1-score = 0.8694, 0.8690, 0.8690, Macro averaging treats both classes equally, reflecting overall balanced model behavior. Weighted average (accounting for class support) for precision, recall, F1-score = 0.8694, 0.8690, 0.8690, the support (sample count) per class and reaffirm consistent performance with respect to the dataset distribution.

The ROC curve of SimpleCNN_Histo model for training dataset is shown in Fig. 4.26. This ROC curve with an AUC of 1.00 signifies that the SimpleCNN_Histo model being evaluated achieves perfect discrimination between the two classes (e.g., Normal vs. OSCC). This means there's a threshold at which the model correctly identifies all positive cases and all negative cases, without any overlap or misclassification.

The SimpleCNN_Histo model demonstrates moderately strong performance in classifying between Normal and OSCC images in the validation dataset. The slightly better recall in the OSCC class is a positive sign for medical diagnostics, as it reduces the likelihood of missing actual cancer cases. However, both classes exhibit some performance trade-offs, and further optimization through hyperparameter tuning, model refinement, or additional training data could help improve generalization. This model, even with an 86.90% accuracy, could be effectively deployed as a preliminary screening tool, potentially flagging cases for further clinical review and reducing manual diagnostic load in oral cancer screening pipelines.

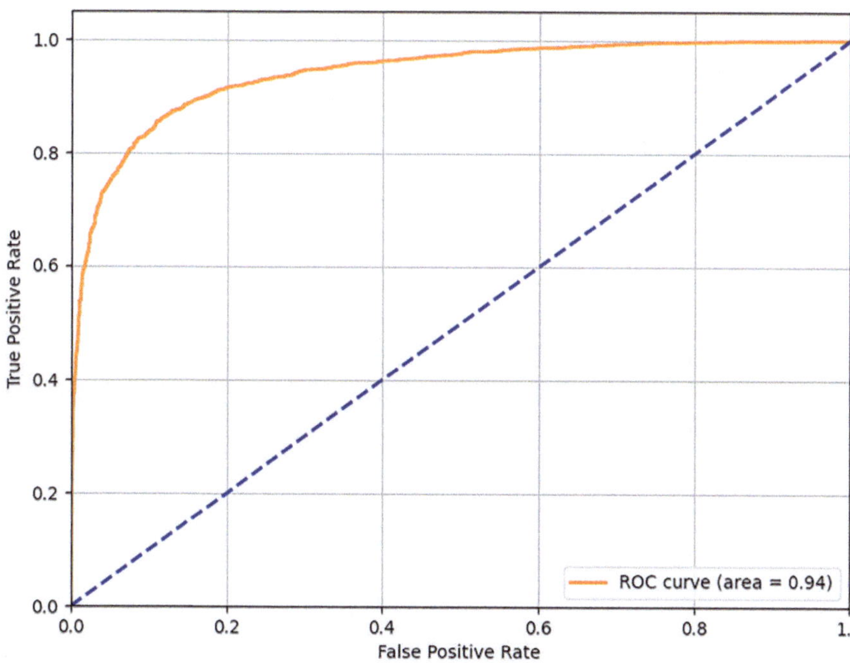

Fig. 4.26 ROC curve for training dataset

4.3.4 Oral Histopathology AI Screening Aid

This section gives the oral histopathology AI screening aid, a specialized application designed to assist in the preliminary screening of histopathological images for Oral Squamous Cell Carcinoma (OSCC). Leveraging a sophisticated SimpleCNN_Histo model trained on a comprehensive dataset of histopathology slides, this tool provides an AI-assisted classification (either "Normal" or "OSCC"). The primary objective is to offer an initial, rapid assessment, thereby potentially streamlining the diagnostic workflow. As shown in Fig. 4.27, the application features a clean interface for image upload.

Figure 4.28 illustrates a sample analysis report with the predicted class and confidence level. It is crucial to underscore that this AI tool is intended solely for informational and assistive purposes and should not, under any circumstances, replace the comprehensive microscopic examination, clinical context, or the final diagnosis made by a qualified and experienced pathologist.

The application offers a straightforward user experience for uploading histopathology images, allowing users to drag and drop files or browse for them, with support for various image formats including JPG, JPEG, PNG, BMP, TIF, and TIFF, up to 200 MB. Upon image submission, the integrated CNN model processes the visual data and presents a clear AI analysis result, including the "Predicted Histopathology Class" and an "AI Confidence Level." This is followed by a "Medical Interpretation & Recommendation" section that provides contextual guidance based on the AI's finding, such as advising continued routine clinical correlation for a "Normal" prediction, or prompt further investigation for any persistent clinical suspicion. This efficient AI-powered screening aims to serve as a valuable initial filter, aiding pathologists and medical professionals in their diligent work.

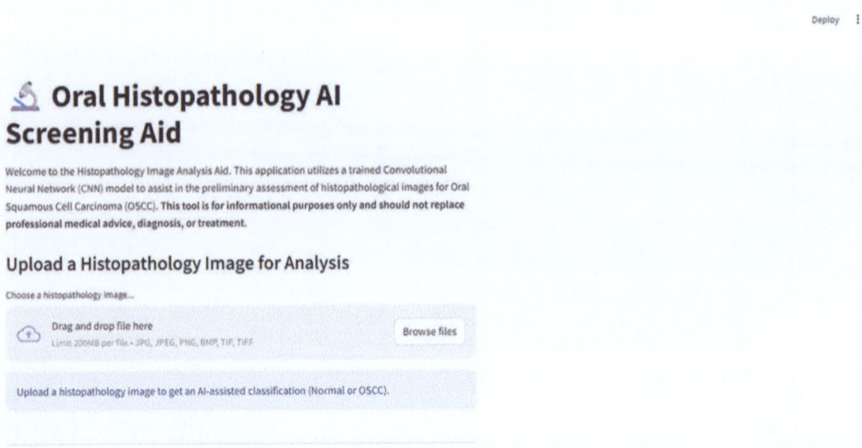

Fig. 4.27 UI of oral histopathology AI screening aid

It is imperative to note the inherent nature and limitations of this tool. As clearly stated within the application's interface, the "Oral Histopathology AI Screening Aid" is developed for advanced informational and research purposes only. It is explicitly not designed to be a diagnostic device and should NOT replace professional medical advice, comprehensive clinical evaluation, diagnostic procedures, or the invaluable judgment of qualified healthcare professionals. Its purpose is to serve as an intelligent assistant, augmenting human expertise in the complex domain of oral cancer assessment.

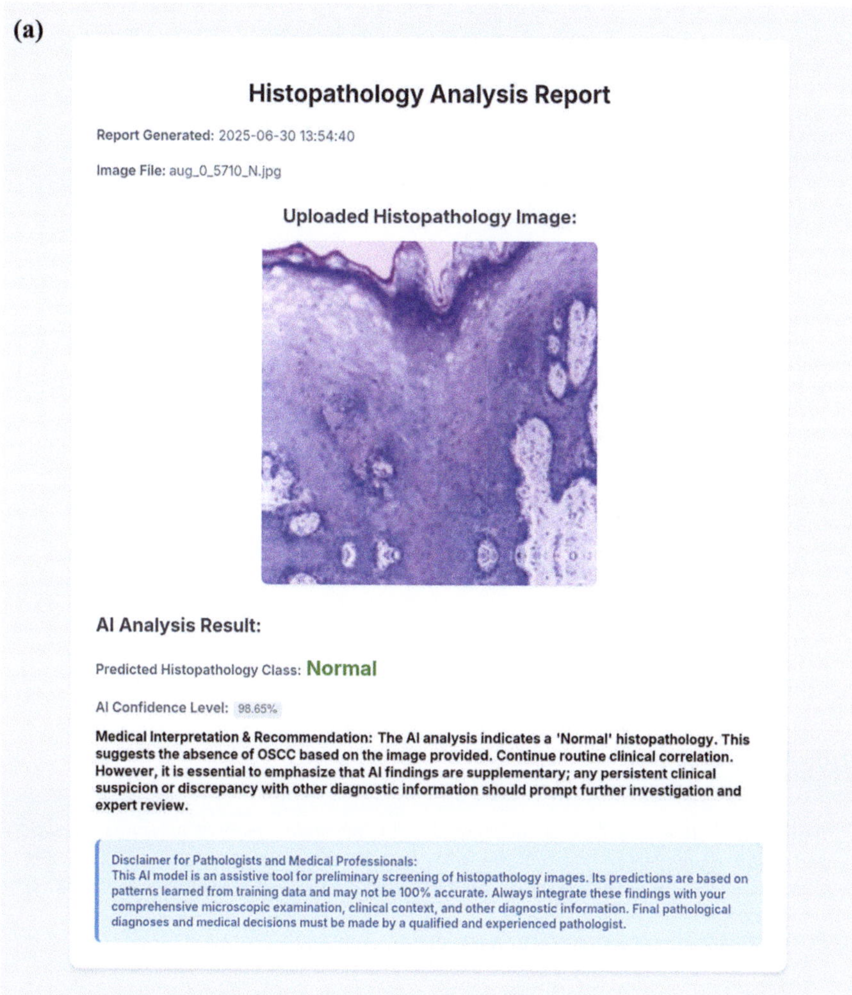

Fig. 4.28 Results generated by oral histopathology AI screening aid (**a**) Case 1 and (**b**) Case 2

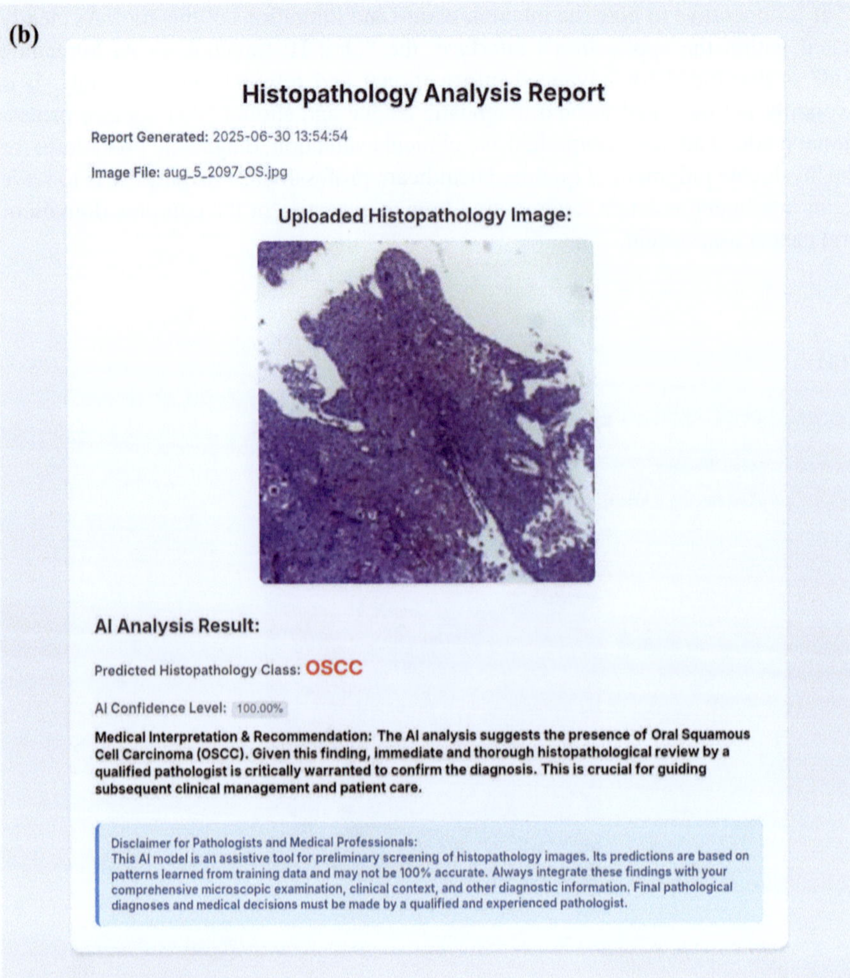

Fig. 4.28 (continued)

References

1. Best, H., & Wolf, C. (2015). Logistic regression. In *The SAGE handbook of regression analysis and causal inference* (pp. 153–171). Sage.
2. Warnakulasuriya, S. (2009). Global epidemiology of oral and oropharyngeal cancer. *Oral Oncology, 45*(4–5), 309–316.
3. Panday, A. (2023). *Oral cancer prediction dataset*. Kaggle. https://www.kaggle.com/datasets/ankushpanday2/oral-cancer-prediction-dataset
4. *Oral cancer dataset*. Retrieved June 2025, from https://www.kaggle.com/datasets/zaidpy/oral-cancer-dataset
5. Rahman, T. Y., et al. (2020). Histopathological imaging database for oral cancer analysis. *Data in Brief, 29*, 105114.

6. *Histopathologic oral cancer detection dataset*. Retrieved June 2025, from https://www.kaggle.com/code/kirollosashraf/histopathologic-oral-cancer-detection
7. Nogueira, M., & Gomes, E. (2025). Histopathological imaging dataset for oral cancer analysis: A study with a data leakage warning. In *Proceedings of the 18th International Joint Conference on Biomedical Engineering Systems and Technologies—Volume 1: Biosignals* (pp. 811–818). SciTePress. https://doi.org/10.5220/0013382100003911

Chapter 5
Multimodal AI for Holistic Oral Cancer Diagnosis and Assessment

The chapter presented the architecture and implementation of a novel multimodal AI system designed to provide a comprehensive and holistic assessment for oral cancer. By integrating analyses from diverse data sources specifically, oral cavity RGB images, histopathology images, and structure patient clinical data, the system aims to overcome the limitations of single-modality diagnostics. Convolutional Neural Networks (CNNs) are employed for robust image feature extraction and classification, while a large language model (LLM) (e.g., OpenAI [1], Google's Gemini [2]) synthesizes insights from all modalities to generate a medically relevant report. This holistic approach promises to enhance the diagnostic accuracy, facilitate earlier detection, and support clinical decision-making, offering a more complete patient profile than individual data streams alone.

This chapter details the development of a conceptual multimodal AI system for oral cancer analysis. We explore the integration of visual data (oral cavity RGB images and histopathology slides) processed by specialized CNNs, alongside structured patient clinical information. The unique contribution lies in using a powerful LLM to synthesize the outputs from these diverse sources, generating a "holistic" narrative that highlights concordances or discordances across findings and offers nuanced clinical recommendations. This approach aims to move beyond simple classification to provide a richer, more interpretable, and clinically relevant assessment, thereby aiding healthcare professionals in their critical decision-making processes.

R. Thanki, S. Shah, *Artificial Intelligence for Early Detection and Diagnosis of Oral Cancer*, Signals and Communication Technology,
https://doi.org/10.1007/978-3-032-05056-4_5

5.1 Background and Related Work

The application of AI in healthcare has seen exponential growth, particularly with the advent of deep learning. Convolutional Neural Networks (CNNs) have emerged as the dominant paradigm for medical image analysis due to their unparalleled ability to learn hierarchical features directly from raw image data. From retinal disease detection to dermatological lesion classification, CNNs have demonstrated human-level (and sometimes superhuman) performance. Transfer learning, where pre-trained CNNs (e.g., VGG, ResNet, EfficientNet) are fine-tuned on smaller medical datasets, has proven especially effective, addressing challenges posed by limited annotated medical images.

While single-modality AI systems are powerful, many medical conditions require information from multiple sources (e.g., imaging, lab tests, patient history, and genomics) for a definitive diagnosis and treatment plan. Multimodal AI seeks to emulate this human physician capability by integrating data from diverse modalities. Early multimodal approaches often involved concatenating features extracted from different data types. More advanced methods utilize specialized fusion techniques, where information from each modality is processed independently and then combined at various levels (early, late, or hybrid fusion) to build a more robust and comprehensive understanding. Examples include combining imaging with genomic data for cancer prognostication or integrating electronic health records with patient wearables.

Large language models, exemplified by models like OpenAI, Google's Gemini, have transformed natural language processing. Their ability to understand, synthesize, and generate human-like text from complex instructions makes them invaluable for tasks requiring contextual reasoning, summarization, and report generation. In medicine, LLMs are being explored for clinical note summarization, answering medical questions, and even assisting in differential diagnosis by integrating vast amounts of medical knowledge. Their application in multimodal settings, where they interpret outputs from other AI models alongside structured data, represents a frontier for generating comprehensive, human-readable medical reports.

5.2 Multimodal AI System for Oral Cancer Analysis

This section details the architecture and components of the proposed AI system for holistic oral cancer assessment.

5.2.1 System Architecture Overview

The system (as shown in Fig. 5.1) is designed as a pipeline that ingests data from three distinct modalities, processes each independently, integrates their findings, and then leverages an LLM for final synthesis.

The basic layers of this system are as follows:

- **Input Layer:**
  - Oral cavity RGB image.
  - Histopathology image.
  - Patient clinical data (CSV).
- **Analysis Layer (Parallel Processing):**
  - **Oral cavity RGB image analysis module:** CNN (e.g., SimpleCNN).
  - **Histopathology image analysis module:** CNN (e.g., SimpleCNN_Histo).
  - **Patient data processing module:** Tabular data extraction/summary.
- **Integration Layer:**
  - Feature fusion/structured prompt generation.
- **Holistic Interpretation Layer:**
  - Large language model (LLM—e.g., Gemini).
- **Output Layer:**
  - Holistic medical report (Textual).

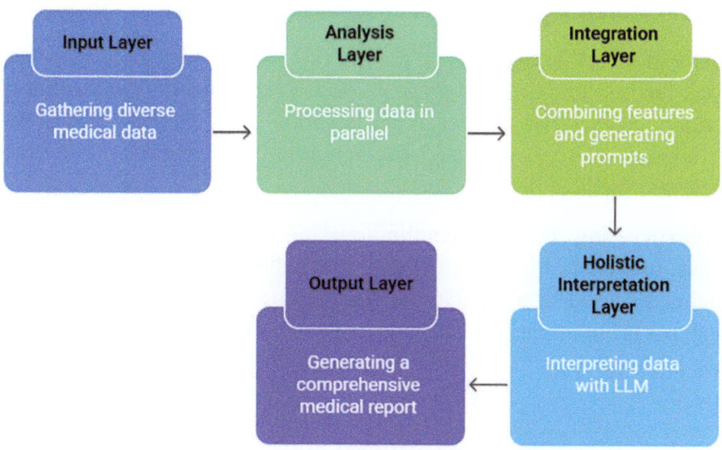

Fig. 5.1 Conceptual architecture of the multimodal oral cancer analysis system

5.2.2 Data Acquisition and Preprocessing

Effective multimodal AI hinges on high-quality and consistently preprocessed data across all modalities.

- **Oral Cavity RGB Images:** These are clinical photographs of the oral cavity.
  - **Acquisition:** Typically captured using standard digital cameras in a clinical setting.
  - **Preprocessing:** Images are resized to uniform (224, 224) pixels to match the input requirements of the CNN model. Pixel values are normalized from the [0, 255] range to [0.0, 1.0] by dividing by 255.0. Data augmentation techniques (e.g., rotation, shifting, zooming, and flipping) are applied during training to enhance model generalization.
- **Oral Histopathology Images:** These are microscopic images of tissue biopsies, typically stained with Hematoxylin and Eosin (H&E).
  - **Acquisition:** Obtained from whole slide scanners, often involving splitting whole slide images (WSIs) into smaller, manageable patches.
  - **Preprocessing:** Like RGB images, histopathology images/patches are resized to consistent (224, 224) pixels and normalized [0.0, 1.0]. Augmentation is also crucial here due to the variability in tissue orientation and staining.
- **Patient Clinical Data (Tabular):** Structured patient information containing relevant clinical parameters.
  - **Acquisition:** Typically, from Electronic Health Records (EHRs) or dedicated patient databases, often exported as CSV files.
  - **Key Features:** For oral cancer assessment, critical features include:

    Demographics: age, gender.
    Risk factors: smoking history (e.g., pack-years), alcohol consumption.
    Lesion characteristics: size (cm), location (e.g., tongue, buccal mucosa), appearance (e.g., ulcerated, erythematous, leukoplakia).
    Relevant medical history.
  - **Preprocessing:** Involves handling missing values, encoding categorical variables, and ensuring consistent data types. Numerical features might be normalized if used by a separate tabular ML model. For LLM integration, these features are summarized into a descriptive text string.

5.2.3 Modality-Specific AI Models

Dedicated CNNs are trained for each image modality to extract relevant features and provide a preliminary classification, forming the "expert opinions" that feed into the LLM.

- **Oral Cavity RGB Image Analysis Model (SimpleCNN Model):** The detailed analysis of this model already covered in Chap. 4. Here, we just provide a summary of the model in context of development for multimodal AI approach.
  - **Objective:** Classify oral cavity images as "No Referral Needed" or "Referral Warranted."
  - **Architecture (Simple CNN):** A sequential CNN model comprising multiple convolutional layers (e.g., 32, 64, 128 filters with 3×3 kernels, ReLU activation), followed by max-pooling layers for dimensionality reduction. A flatten layer connects to dense layers (e.g., 512 units with ReLU) and a final output sigmoid layer for binary classification. Dropout layers (e.g., 0.5) are included for regularization.
  - **Training:** Trained on a balanced dataset of oral cavity RGB images (e.g., 30,000 images, 15,000 per class), split into 80% training and 20% validation. Optimized with Adam, using binary cross-entropy loss, over 10 epochs.
  - **Output:** A probability score between 0 and 1, interpreted as the likelihood of "No Referral Needed" or "Referral Warranted."
- **Histopathology Image Analysis Model (SimpleCNN_Histo):** The detailed analysis of this model already covered in Chap. 4. Here, we just provide a summary of the model in context of development for multimodal AI.
  - **Objective:** Classify histopathology images as "Normal" or "OSCC."
  - **Architecture:** Similar simple CNN architecture as the RGB model, allowing for consistent input processing.
  - **Training:** Trained on a balanced dataset of histopathology images/patches (e.g., 30,000 images; 15,000 per class), split into 80% training and 20% validation. Optimized with Adam, using binary cross-entropy loss, over 10 epochs.
  - **Output:** A probability score between 0 and 1, interpreted as the likelihood of "Normal" or "OSCC."

5.2.4 Data Integration and Feature Fusion

The outputs from the modality-specific models are integrated to create a unified input for the LLM. This involves translating numerical predictions and structured tabular data into a coherent textual format.

- CNN predictions (predicted class name, confidence percentage) are converted into descriptive sentences.
- Key patient clinical data points from the CSV are extracted and summarized into a natural language string.
- Crucially, the original images (as Base64 encoded byte streams) are passed alongside textual descriptions as multimodal input to the Gemini LLM. This allows Gemini to perform visual reasoning in addition to text understanding.

5.2.5 Holistic Interpretation Using Large Language Models

LLMs (e.g., OpenAI, Google Gemini) serve as the central intelligence for generating holistic assessment.

- **Input to LLM:** A carefully crafted prompt containing:
  - System instructions (role: specialized AI assistant).
  - Detailed findings from the oral cavity RGB image analysis.
  - Detailed findings from the histopathology image analysis.
  - Summary of patient clinical data.
  - The raw RGB and histopathology image data as multimodal elements.
  - Specific instructions on the desired output structure (summary, concordance analysis, overall assessment, recommendations, and disclaimer).
- **LLM's Function:** LLM processes this complex, multimodal input to:
  - **Synthesize Information:** Combine insights from visual and textual data.
  - **Identify Concordance/Discordance:** Determine if the findings from different modalities align (e.g., RGB suggests referral, Histo suggests OSCC) or conflict (e.g., RGB suggests no referral, Histo suggests OSCC).
  - **Contextualize Findings:** Interpret results within the broader clinical context provided by patient data.
  - **Generate Comprehensive Narrative:** Produce a human-readable, structured report that mirrors clinical reasoning.
  - **Provide Actionable Recommendations:** Suggest next steps for patient management based on the holistic view.
- **Justification for LLM:** The LLM's ability to handle ambiguous inputs, perform nuanced reasoning, and generate coherent, structured text makes it ideal for integrating disparate data points into a single, clinically valuable narrative, far beyond what simple rule-based systems could achieve.

5.2.6 Implementation Details

The multimodal AI system is implemented using Python, leveraging robust and widely adopted frameworks.

- **Programming Language:** Python (version 3.8+).
- **Machine Learning Framework:** TensorFlow 2.x/Keras for building, training, and deploying CNN models.
- **Data Processing:** Pandas library for efficient handling and summarization of tabular (CSV) patient data. PIL (Pillow) for image loading and preprocessing.

- **User Interface:** Streamlit for creating an interactive web application, allowing users to upload data and view results easily. Streamlit's st.cache_resource is used to cache loaded models for efficient app performance.
- **Multimodal LLM Integration:** Google's google-generative AI library is used to interact with the Gemini API. Asynchronous programming (asyncio) is employed for non-blocking API calls within the Streamlit environment.
- **API Key Management:** The appropriate API key is securely loaded from environment variables to avoid hardcoding credentials.
- **Model Storage:** Trained CNN models are saved in the H5 format for easy loading.
- **Output:** The analysis report is displayed directly in the Streamlit interface and can also be downloaded as a static HTML file for offline viewing and record-keeping, formatted to medical standards.

5.3 Multimodal Oral Cancer Assistant (MOCA) Agent

This section introduces the MOCA (Multimodal Oral Cancer Assistant) agent, a sophisticated application designed to leverage the power of discriminative AI (CNNs) and generative AI (Gemini AI) for a comprehensive and integrated assessment of oral cancer. This aims to empower clinicians with deeper insights into earlier detection and more precise treatment planning. As depicted in the accompanying interface (as shown in Fig. 5.2), this advanced tool distinguishes itself by integrating multimodal data, specifically drawing insights from oral cavity RGB images, oral histopathology images, and patient clinical data. The overarching goal is to move beyond isolated data analysis, providing a holistic understanding of a patient's condition for more informed clinical decision-making.

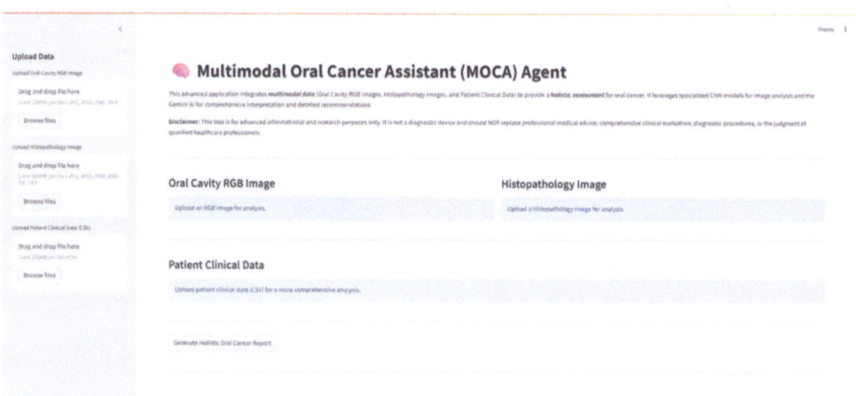

Fig. 5.2 UI of Multimodal Oral Cancer Assistant (MOCA) agent before data uploaded

The application's robust capabilities are underpinned by a dual-component AI architecture. It utilizes specialized Convolutional Neural Network (CNN) models for the intricate analysis of both oral cavity RGB images and oral histopathology slides, extracting critical visual features indicative of cancerous or pre-cancerous conditions. These visual insights, combined with structured patient clinical data, are then fed into a powerful Large Language Model (LLM), such as Gemini AI. The LLM's role is to perform a comprehensive interpretation of all integrated data, synthesizing disparate information into coherent, detailed recommendations and a holistic diagnostic overview. The user interface is designed for intuitive data submission, featuring dedicated "Upload Data" sections on the left panel. Users can easily upload:

- **Oral Cavity RGB Image:** Facilitating the input of photographic images of the oral cavity, supporting formats like JPG, JPEG, PNG, and BMP, with a file size limit of 200 MB/file.
- **Histopathology Image:** Allowing the submission of high-resolution histopathological slides, accommodating formats such as JPG, JPEG, PNG, BMP, TIF, and TIFF, also with a 200 MB/file limit.
- **Patient Clinical Data (CSV):** Enabling the upload of structured patient information in CSV format, crucial for providing context to the image analyses, with a 200 MB/file limit.

Upon successful data upload across the required modalities (as shown in Fig. 5.3), the system allows the user to initiate the analysis process by clicking the "Generate Holistic Oral Cancer Report" button. This action triggers the integrated AI pipeline, culminating in a detailed holistic oral cancer report. This report is generated as an HTML-compatible textual format, allowing for a clearly structured output with headings, organized sections, and improved readability, designed for easy viewing within a web browser or similar digital document viewer. As shown in the sample report (as shown in Fig. 5.4), the report provides a comprehensive

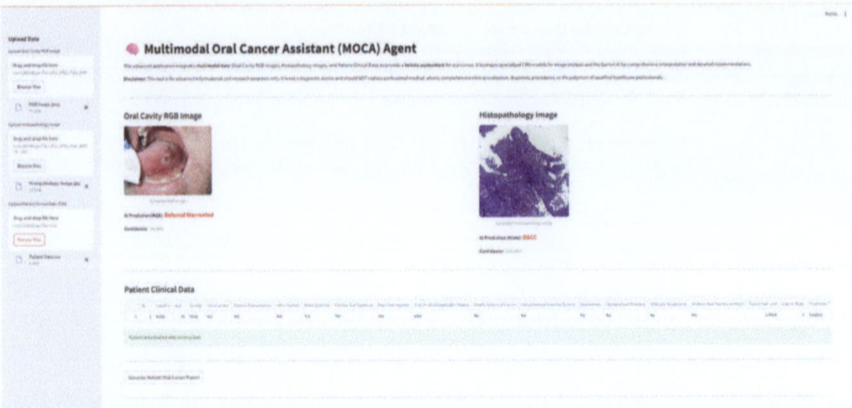

Fig. 5.3 UI of Multimodal Oral Cancer Assistant (MOCA) agent after data uploaded

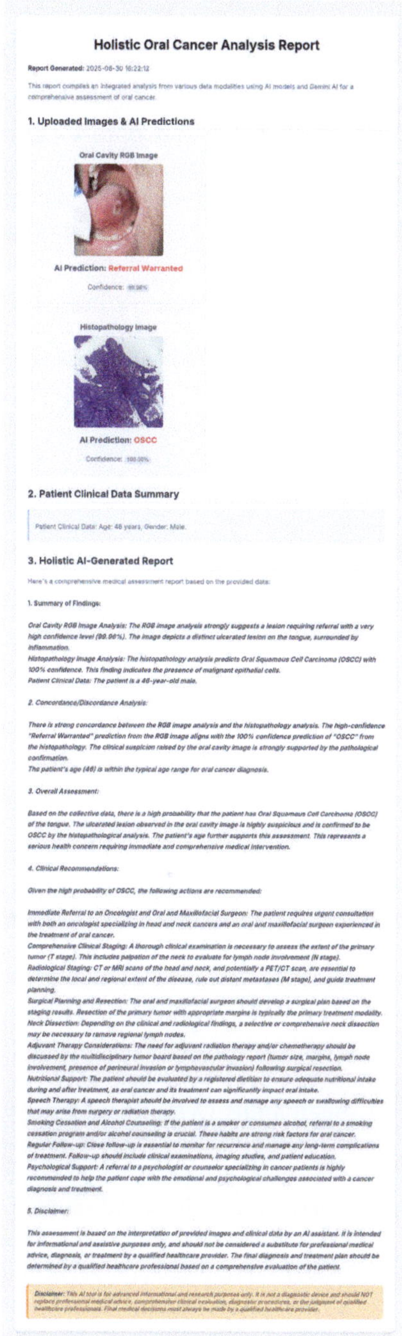

Holistic Oral Cancer Analysis Report

Report Generated: 2025-08-30 16:22:12

This report compiles an integrated analysis from various data modalities using AI models and Gemini AI for a comprehensive assessment of oral cancer.

1. Uploaded Images & AI Predictions

Oral Cavity RGB Image

AI Prediction: Referral Warranted

Confidence: 99.96%

Histopathology Image

AI Prediction: OSCC

Confidence: 100.00%

2. Patient Clinical Data Summary

Patient Clinical Data: Age: 46 years, Gender: Male.

3. Holistic AI-Generated Report

Here's a comprehensive medical assessment report based on the provided data:

1. Summary of Findings:

Oral Cavity RGB Image Analysis: The RGB image analysis strongly suggests a lesion requiring referral with a very high confidence level (99.96%). The image depicts a distinct ulcerated lesion on the tongue, surrounded by inflammation.
Histopathology Image Analysis: The histopathology analysis predicts Oral Squamous Cell Carcinoma (OSCC) with 100% confidence. This finding indicates the presence of malignant epithelial cells.
Patient Clinical Data: The patient is a 46-year-old male.

2. Concordance/Discordance Analysis:

There is strong concordance between the RGB image analysis and the histopathology analysis. The high-confidence "Referral Warranted" prediction from the RGB image aligns with the 100% confidence prediction of "OSCC" from the histopathology. The clinical suspicion raised by the oral cavity image is strongly supported by the pathological confirmation.
The patient's age (46) is within the typical age range for oral cancer diagnosis.

3. Overall Assessment:

Based on the collective data, there is a high probability that the patient has Oral Squamous Cell Carcinoma (OSCC) of the tongue. The ulcerated lesion observed in the oral cavity image is highly suspicious and is confirmed to be OSCC by the histopathological analysis. The patient's age further supports this assessment. This represents a serious health concern requiring immediate and comprehensive medical intervention.

4. Clinical Recommendations:

Given the high probability of OSCC, the following actions are recommended:

Immediate Referral to an Oncologist and Oral and Maxillofacial Surgeon: The patient requires urgent consultation with both an oncologist specializing in head and neck cancers and an oral and maxillofacial surgeon experienced in the treatment of oral cancer.
Comprehensive Clinical Staging: A thorough clinical examination is necessary to assess the extent of the primary tumor (T stage). This includes palpation of the neck to evaluate for lymph node involvement (N stage).
Radiological Staging: CT or MRI scans of the head and neck, and potentially a PET/CT scan, are essential to determine the local and regional extent of the disease, rule out distant metastases (M stage), and guide treatment planning.
Surgical Planning and Resection: The oral and maxillofacial surgeon should develop a surgical plan based on the staging results. Resection of the primary tumor with appropriate margins is typically the primary treatment modality.
Neck Dissection: Depending on the clinical and radiological findings, a selective or comprehensive neck dissection may be necessary to remove regional lymph nodes.
Adjuvant Therapy Considerations: The need for adjuvant radiation therapy and/or chemotherapy should be discussed by the multidisciplinary tumor board based on the pathology report (tumor size, margins, lymph node involvement, presence of perineural invasion or lymphovascular invasion) following surgical resection.
Nutritional Support: The patient should be evaluated by a registered dietitian to ensure adequate nutritional intake during and after treatment, as oral cancer and its treatment can significantly impact oral intake.
Speech Therapy: A speech therapist should be involved to assess and manage any speech or swallowing difficulties that may arise from surgery or radiation therapy.
Smoking Cessation and Alcohol Counseling: If the patient is a smoker or consumes alcohol, referral to a smoking cessation program and/or alcohol counseling is crucial. These habits are strong risk factors for oral cancer.
Regular Follow-up: Close follow-up is essential to monitor for recurrence and manage any long-term complications of treatment. Follow-up should include clinical examinations, imaging studies, and patient education.
Psychological Support: A referral to a psychologist or counselor specializing in cancer patients is highly recommended to help the patient cope with the emotional and psychological challenges associated with a cancer diagnosis and treatment.

5. Disclaimer:

This assessment is based on the interpretation of provided images and clinical data by an AI assistant. It is intended for informational and assistive purposes only, and should not be considered a substitute for professional medical advice, diagnosis, or treatment by a qualified healthcare provider. The final diagnosis and treatment plan should be determined by a qualified healthcare professional based on a comprehensive evaluation of the patient.

Disclaimer: *This AI tool is for advanced informational and research purposes only. It is not a diagnostic device and should NOT replace professional medical advice, comprehensive clinical evaluation, diagnostic procedures, or the judgment of qualified healthcare professionals. Final medical decisions must always be made by a qualified healthcare provider.*

Fig. 5.4 Results generated by Multimodal Oral Cancer Assistant (MOCA) agent

summary of findings, potential diagnoses, and actionable recommendations derived from the multimodal analysis.

It is imperative to note the inherent nature and limitations of this tool. As clearly stated within the application's interface, the "Multimodal Oral Cancer Assistant (MOCA) Agent" is developed for advanced informational and research purposes only. It is explicitly not designed to be a diagnostic device and should NOT replace professional medical advice, comprehensive clinical evaluation, diagnostic procedures, or the invaluable judgment of qualified healthcare professionals. Its purpose is to serve as an intelligent assistant, augmenting human expertise in the complex domain of oral cancer assessment.

This chapter has demonstrated the feasibility and potential of a multimodal AI system for holistic oral cancer assessment. By combining insights from oral cavity RGB images, oral histopathology images, and patient clinical data using specialized CNNs and a powerful LLM, the proposed system aims to provide a more comprehensive, integrated, and clinically actionable diagnostic aid. This holistic approach has the potential to significantly enhance early detection strategies and improve patient management in the fight against oral cancer. Future work will focus on further enhancing the system's robustness, accuracy, and clinical utility:

- **Larger and More Diverse Datasets:** Expanding the training datasets for all modalities to include more diverse patient populations, image acquisition protocols, and disease variations (e.g., different grades of dysplasia, benign lesions for differential diagnosis).
- **Advanced Feature Fusion:** Exploring more sophisticated multimodal fusion techniques beyond simple concatenation or sequential prompting, potentially involving attention mechanisms or multimodal transformers.
- **Quantifying Concordance:** Developing quantitative metrics to assess and report the degree of concordance or discordance between modality-specific findings, providing a more objective measure for clinicians.
- **Integration with EHRs:** Developing secure and compliant interfaces for direct, real-time integration with Electronic Health Records (EHRs) to automate data ingestion and streamline clinical workflows.
- **Formal Clinical Validation:** Conducting prospective clinical trials to rigorously validate the system's performance, impact on diagnostic accuracy, and patient outcomes in real-world settings.
- **Explainability (XAI):** Enhancing the explainability features beyond the LLM's narrative, perhaps by integrating visual saliency maps (e.g., Grad-CAM) directly into the holistic report to highlight regions of interest in the images.
- **Feedback Loops for Continuous Learning:** Implementing mechanisms for clinicians to provide feedback on AI assessments, which can then be used to continuously refine and improve the models.
- **Scalability and Deployment:** Optimizing the application for cloud deployment and higher scalability to serve multiple users or integrate into larger healthcare IT infrastructures.

References

1. OpenAI. (2024). *OpenAI API documentation*. https://openai.com/api
2. Google. (2024). *Gemini API documentation*. https://ai.google.dev/gemini-api

Index

R. Thanki, S. Shah, *Artificial Intelligence for Early Detection and Diagnosis of Oral Cancer*, Signals and Communication Technology,
https://doi.org/10.1007/978-3-032-05056-4

MIX
Papier aus verantwortungsvollen Quellen
Paper from responsible sources
FSC® C105338

If you have any concerns about our products, you can contact us on
ProductSafety@springernature.com

In case Publisher is established outside the EU, the EU authorized representative is:
Springer Nature Customer Service Center GmbH
Europaplatz 3, 69115 Heidelberg, Germany

Printed by Libri Plureos GmbH
in Hamburg, Germany